"Case studies are making a comeback in neuropsychology, especially for teaching. They are memorable and come closer to teaching the skill of neuropsychology than abstract knowledge can. Mistakes are especially memorable, but also shameful and so they are understudied. I salute the courage and wisdom of these thoughtful and skilled authors in modeling for all of us how to learn from our mistakes in assessment and treatment. If, through their example, we can all learn to focus on the lessons of our mistakes, we may be able to improve and accelerate neuropsychological training."

Ted Judd, *Clinical Neuropsychologist and Cross-Cultural Specialist, Associate Professor Seattle Pacific University*

"A decidedly human and entertaining account of some of the mistakes we can make while learning and practicing our profession. A very useful resource for training and expanding our development."

George P. Prigatano, Ph.D., *Emeritus Chairman of Clinical Neuropsychology, Barrow Neurological Institute*

Mistakes in Clinical Neuropsychology

This innovative book uses a case-based approach to discuss mistakes made in the practice of clinical neuropsychology to form a helpful tool in the training of early career clinicians. By allowing readers space for critical reflection during clinical practice, the book teaches competency in clinical neuropsychology, through the examination of errors as a central part of the learning process.

The core of this book is a diverse series of mistakes, each embedded as a patient narrative. Each chapter is based around an example error, typically one that was made, by the authors, as early career clinicians. Early chapters focus on mistakes in neuropsychological assessment and the diagnostic process. Later chapters focus on errors in rehabilitation and management. Each chapter is framed to reflect the situational context, for example the role of history, what constitutes normal performance, the way that complex tasks rely on foundational skills, or the treatment of patients with dysexecutive impairment. Towards the end of each chapter, there is reflection on the nature of each error type. As such, each chapter follows the structure SEER (Situation, Example, Error and Reflection), helping the reader to imagine the situation around the mistake, its nature and relevance. The book especially emphasises small phrases of insight (axioms or gnomes) that are widely used by experienced clinicians.

This is valuable reading for students of clinical neuropsychology, occupational therapy and speech and language therapy as well as professionals in these fields such as neurologists, psychiatrists and other rehabilitation therapists. It is especially appropriate for those in the earlier stages of their career in clinical neuropsychology, or in related disciplines which involve the assessment and treatment of patients with neurological disorders that impair cognition or disrupt the regulation of emotion. However, experienced clinicians will also find that it includes interesting insights to improve their practice.

Oliver Turnbull is a neuropsychologist and clinical psychologist, with an interest in emotion, especially as related to emotion regulation, memory, decision-making, false beliefs and the neuroscience of psychotherapy. He is Professor at Bangor University in Wales, UK, where he is also Deputy Vice Chancellor.

Rudi Coetzer is an Honorary Professor in the School of Human and Behavioural Sciences at Bangor University, and in the Faculty of Medicine, Health & Life Science, Swansea University. He worked in the National Health Service for 20 years as Consultant Neuropsychologist and Head of Service before taking up the role of Clinical Director for a UK brain injury rehabilitation charity during 2021.

Christian Salas is a clinical neuropsychologist and psychoanalytic psychotherapist. He is Associate Lecturer at the Center for Human Neuroscience and Neuropsychology and Director of the Clinical Neuropsychology Unit (Diego Portales University). His work focuses on understanding emotional and personality changes after brain injury and how psychoanalytic tools can be adapted to facilitate socio-emotional adjustment and well-being.

Mistakes in Clinical Neuropsychology

Learning from a Case-based Approach

Oliver Turnbull, Rudi Coetzer and Christian Salas

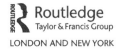

Routledge
Taylor & Francis Group

LONDON AND NEW YORK

Designed cover image: Oliver Turnbull

First published 2023
by Routledge
4 Park Square, Milton Park, Abingdon, Oxon OX14 4RN

and by Routledge
605 Third Avenue, New York, NY 10158

Routledge is an imprint of the Taylor & Francis Group, an informa business

British Library Cataloguing-in-Publication Data
A catalogue record for this book is available from the British Library

ISBN: 9781032292670 (hbk)
ISBN: 9781032292663 (pbk)
ISBN: 9781003300748 (ebk)

DOI: 10.4324/9781003300748

Typeset in Bembo
by Apex CoVantage, LLC

In the early part of my career, I made an assumption that human knowledge developed in a steady progression building on what went before, that we gradually, or more rapidly at times, eradicate our mistakes. Experience, as you know, proves this to be false and many of the battles have to be fought over and over again.

Kevin Walsh (1992) Some Gnomes Worth Knowing, p.119–120.

Contents

Foreword

It is a truism that we should learn from our mistakes. However, the fact that we often find ourselves making the same mistakes again and again suggests that we may not be terribly good at reflecting on our bad decisions. Alas, this is probably true in many aspects of our lives, including in our work as neuropsychologists!

As this impressive book makes clear, one of the reasons is that clinical neuropsychology is a very complex area of work. Difficult as it is to accept, none of us knows all the things that we would like to know.

The book also makes it clear that it can be hard to admit when we have made an error, even – perhaps especially – to ourselves. It is doubly hard to admit our mistake to someone else, especially if that person is a colleague, and if the error involves your work with a patient. But this book is a wonderful illustration of why it is so important that, throughout our careers, we take time to stop and reflect, whenever we notice that we have made a mistake. We really do need to learn from these opportunities.

This book not only prompts us to think about our own errors, but – inspiringly – we also have the chance to learn from the mistakes made by colleagues who *themselves* have learned from their mistakes. In this book, Oliver, Rudi and Christian, who I've known for many years, share their learning experiences with us. They are some of the wisest clinical neuropsychologists I know, and it's clear to me that some of their wisdom has come from a willingness to think deeply about their work, including their mistakes.

If you are reading this Foreword wondering whether to read the rest of the book, my advice is . . . don't hesitate. You are in for a treat, and you will find the cases fascinating. I found some very useful insights into the practice of clinical neuropsychology, including issues about clinical work that are important, but seldom discussed. All of them are things that early career clinicians will find especially helpful, and the book will be recommended reading for trainees on our clinical neuropsychology programme.

I especially enjoyed the structure of the chapters: a case presented, an error explained and reflection on what can be learned. The storytelling in each case is gripping. Knowing that the book is about mistakes prompts you (or at least it did for me) to play the game of trying to anticipate the error, but of course it is rarely predictable! Oliver, Rudi and Christian are wonderful storytellers. Importantly, the cases are described in enough detail that clinicians will easily recognise the types of patient being presented. This makes it easy to think about one's own cases, and indeed one's own mistakes!

I was also delighted to see that there are chapters that focus on neuropsychological rehabilitation, and not simply on diagnostic assessment. The chapters also cover a range of conditions and cognitive domains, and indeed a range of contexts, including the topical issue of work in under-resourced service settings. Given the complexity of neuropsychological test interpretation, and the huge range of potential pathologies, it is unsurprising that mistakes are made in assessment. But the inclusion of rehabilitation vividly reminds us that treatment and management are also complex processes, and that we need to learn from our mistakes there too.

Almost all of the chapters are illustrated with compelling individual cases. However, in an interesting twist, one chapter focuses on a group-based intervention for people recovering from brain injury. I enjoyed the change in perspective very much. Rather than a simple focus on mistakes, the nuanced emphasis is on lessons learned from unexpected findings in running the intervention. I suspect that these lessons will resonate with clinicians working in rehabilitation.

The book also draws skilfully on the power of gnomes. Not the diminutive goblins who guard earth's hidden treasures (and bedeck many an English garden). But rather the aphorisms passed on by other, wise, neuropsychologists, such as Dr Kevin Walsh. The gnomes succinctly, and charmingly, sum up important lessons that we should all carry to our clinical practice. They are all the more memorable for being bite-sized pieces of wisdom.

This book is going to make it easier for all of us, no matter our level of clinical experience, to acknowledge our mistakes. In turn, this will improve our clinical practice, and that must be a very good thing for our profession.

Now dive in and enjoy this unique and fascinating book.

Professor Jon Evans
Professor of Clinical Neuropsychology
Programme Director for Clinical Neuropsychology Training Programmes
University of Glasgow
Incoming President of the International Neuropsychological Society
October 2022

Preface

'In the early part of my career, I made an assumption . . . that we gradually . . . eradicate our mistakes'.

—*Kevin Walsh (1992) Some Gnomes Worth Knowing, p. 119*

Why should we write a book about *mistakes* made in the practice of clinical neuropsychology? Mistakes? Of all things? Why not focus on the positive? Our response takes two forms: one educational and one emotional.

First is the educational gap. Clinicians agree that mistakes are important. Supervision is there, in large part, to help identify and resolve errors in diagnosis and treatment. And the question of errors, and avoiding them, is a repeated theme in feedback from clinical trainees about supervision (Stucky et al., 2010). In addition, every clinician will have made mistakes, especially early in their careers. We suspect that many clinicians will have made some of the mistakes identified in this book.

Paradoxically, however, those very mistakes are *neither* a common topic of discussion during supervision (Shultz et al., 2014) nor do they commonly appear in papers or textbooks on clinical neuropsychology. Given that people agree that mistakes *should* be discussed, this is an important issue. The final chapter of the book discusses this problem in more detail. Because mistakes are inevitable, they are critical to identify, and they are useful learning opportunities. As that final chapter suggests, mistakes should be *appreciated*. Nevertheless, we remain surprised at how little space has been dedicated to mistakes in the supervision literature.

This is especially surprising in the field of psychology, rather than (say) engineering or biology. All good practitioner psychologists should know that honest acknowledgement of failure is the key to improvement. However, practitioner psychologists also know that acknowledgement of failure comes with emotional consequences. Recognising your errors is not especially common, and having them pointed out is painful and difficult to bear – the pathway towards denial and other defences (see Turnbull & Salas, 2017; Turnbull et al., 2014, for a review of the neuropsychology). A readable account of this issue can be found in Tavris and Aronson's (2008) charmingly titled *Mistakes were made (but not by me).* It is so much easier to focus on the mistakes of others, yet so hard to acknowledge them in ourselves.

This, then, is the emotional justification of this book. Denying a truth, just because it feels bad, is no way to develop as a clinician or as a scientist. Also, however painful, it cannot be denied that mistakes – and the narrative surrounding mistakes – are an excellent teaching tool. Education, wrapped around a personalised anecdote, is often more memorable – probably because the telling of a good story is a skill, and historically crucial in knowledge transfer. Indeed, before modern medicine, writing accurate and perceptive case reports was always a highly valued skill (Code et al., 1996, 2003). Luria's two case-study books (Luria, 1968, 1972), for example, remain some of his most influential and cited works: examples of what he called 'romantic science', and a tradition that fortunately lives on (see Sacks, 1990).

Many of the classic cases in neuropsychology continue to inform clinical practice – especially for the disorders which they represent: Broca's Leborgne (or Tan) for aphasia, HM for amnesia, Phineas Gage for self-regulation and Luria's Zazetsky for his many visuo-spatial impairments. Thus, while modern neuroscience continues to dazzle, with new gadgets and techniques for data analysis, we are also enthusiastic to preserve the art of the case report (see Coetzer & Balchin, 2014, p. 8). We can still learn much through this neglected skill in clinical neuropsychology.

Not least for reasons of memorability. At least in our experience, it is worryingly common to wade through a technical paper, and yet remember little of it a week later. But a narrative well told, a message threaded through a personal story, has far more power to resonate for weeks and years. Because, as Oliver Sacks (1987) noted, stories of patients with brain injury can resemble classical fables and tales, where average human beings become archetypical figures: heroes, victims, martyrs and warriors. Famously, Sacks wrote (admittedly some 40 years ago) that 'Neuropsychology is admirable, but it excludes the *psyche* – it excludes the experiencing, active, living "I"' (Sacks, 1984, p. 184). The case report is, therefore, one important way that the psyche can be given its rightful place in our field.

This aspect of neuropsychological case reports, then, is well established: patients who are somehow 'champions' for the disorders which they represent, iconic for their specific category of aphasia, apraxia and agnosia. However, we believe that the case report can also be a vehicle for understanding the *process* by which clinicians explore, and attempt to understand, disorders. Process is the key to the hypothesis-driven detective work that is at the heart of clinical neuropsychology. When should you ask those extra questions about family background when taking a history? When should you not believe the result of a test, and why should that make you choose another one? When should you follow the rules of test administration, and when should you adapt them? The case report seems a fruitful way to address this difficult problem of decisions and mistakes, because it can place the reader at the centre of a personalised drama, as we look over a shoulder at the trainee's journey.

While we are speaking about memorable things, writing this book has helped us realise that there are a few classic neuropsychological phrases that have echoed in our ears across the decades, bringing to mind a critical issue. Often, we discovered, this was a phrase from the legendary Kevin Walsh. Our favourite is his wonderfully insightful: 'There is . . . no such thing as a neuropsychological test' (Walsh, 1992, p. 130). We have a chapter dedicated to the issue,[1] because understanding the problems that lie behind a 'neuropsychological' test helps avoid a key pitfall in the field. But we remain in awe that it took one of us (OT) an entire chapter to make clear what Walsh sums up in a few words of angry poetry.[2]

The heart of this book is a diverse series of mistakes, each embedded in a chapter, often based around our experiences as trainees and early career clinicians, sometimes decades ago. Most are themed around assessment, with some on rehabilitation. We have worked hard to retain patient (and supervisor) anonymity. Indeed, some cases are amalgams, or even adaptations, of situations and challenges we have encountered. Typically, we experienced these cases directly, but sometimes indirectly through colleagues' sharing of experiences, for which we are grateful.

Notably, each chapter is structured in four phases. We frame the case in an opening section (headed Situation) which discusses the generic problem that the chapter will cover. We then present the clinical case (Example), as it was experienced by the trainee, including the logic of developing a hypothesis, thinking about why this or that approach was selected, and some narrative about patient performance. Perhaps you will read this section the way some people watch horror films: wanting to tell the character 'No . . . don't walk down that dark path!', or 'Why can't you *see* it . . . it's right there, for heaven's sake!'? The third section (and the most painful to write) was that on the mistake (Error). We confess that writing these sections, re-experiencing feedback from a supervisor, did prompt difficult flash-backs, though fortunately they stayed on the correct side of PTSD. Finally, we offer some lessons learned (Reflection).

In our final chapter of the book, we spend some time thinking about the issue of errors in more detail. We consider the principal causes of mistakes, themed around growing your knowledge base, avoiding over-reliance on a single source of information, and how best to manage and develop your intuition. We hope that this last chapter will offer some guidance on how we might gradually build expertise, especially when used in conjunction with the examples in the central chapters.

In writing this book, we have realised that we, and our colleagues, have perhaps learned as much through our failings as we have from our successes. Indeed, we wonder whether, in the career of the average clinical neuropsychologist, this pattern might be more common than we want to admit. Perhaps understandably (as we discussed earlier), nobody tends to talk much about mistakes, or – heaven forbid – formally present their 'best' mistakes at conferences! But after several decades of involvement in clinical neuropsychology, we were also surprised to see that no one appeared to write about this topic – or at the very least we have been unable to find such a book. One does discover a few mentions of 'pitfalls' in a book chapter or paper, but nothing exclusively devoted to 'getting it wrong'. However, it is interesting that the idea of systematically looking at cases that fail, or paying attention to common mistakes that occur in the therapeutic process, has been used as a source of insight in neighbouring disciplines, such as psychoanalytic psychotherapy (Casement, 2002; Goldberg, 2012; Reppen & Schulman, 2001). Regardless, this appears to be the first systematic appearance of the 'mistake' theme in clinical neuropsychology.

Finally, we would especially like to thank the patients with whom we have had the privilege of spending time, the colleagues we have worked with and the students who have kept us on our toes. And, of course, we would also like to thank the clinician-teacher-supervisors from whom we learned so much over the course of many years. We thank you for being gentle with our errors.

Oliver Turnbull, Bangor, Cymru/Wales, UK
Rudi Coetzer, Bangor, Cymru/Wales, UK
Christian Salas, Santiago, Chile

Notes

1 Our book cover is also linked to this theme. We even considered adding a subtitle to the Block Design image, to read: '*This is not a neuropsychological test*'. It would then be a playful nod to the famous Renee Magritte painting: *This is not a pipe*. This painting itself has a rich history in neuropsychology, given that a hat-themed version of the Magritte was on the original (1984) cover of Oliver Sacks' *The man who mistook his wife for a hat*, as a reference to Sacks' story about prosopagnosia.

2 Walsh was fond of these clinical pearls of wisdom, where a highlight is his insightful paper: *Some gnomes worth knowing*. By 'gnomes', Walsh of course means axioms or aphorisms, rather than garden ornaments (Walsh, 1992, p. 119). Indeed, the term is derived from the same Greek term 'gnosis' (knowledge) from which neuropsychology derives the term agnosia. Walsh used these short phrases often, and to great effect, and we have cited several examples across our book.

References

Casement, P. (2002). *Learning from our mistakes: Beyond dogma in psychoanalysis and psychotherapy*. Guilford Press.

Code, C., Wallesch, C.-W., Joanette, Y., & Roch, A. (1996). *Classic cases in neuropsychology*. Psychology Press.

Code, C., Wallesch, C.-W., Joanette, Y., & Roch, A. (2003). *Classic cases in neuropsychology*. Psychology Press.

Coetzer, R., & Balchin, R. (2014). *Working with brain injury: A primer for psychologists working in under-resourced settings*. Psychology Press.

Goldberg, A. (2012). *The analysis of failure: An investigation of failed cases in psychoanalysis and psychotherapy*. Routledge.

Luria, A. (1968). *The mind of a mnemonist: A little book about a vast memory*. Harvard University Press.

Luria, A. (1972). *The man with a shattered world: The history of a brain wound*. Harvard University Press.

Reppen, J., & Schulman, M. (2001). *Failures in psychoanalytic treatment*. Intl Universities Press.

Sacks, O. (1984). *A leg to stand on*. Picador.

Sacks, O. (1987). *The man who mistook his wife for a hat and other clinical tales*. Harper Perennial.

Sacks, O. (1990). Luria and 'romantic science'. In E. Goldberg (Ed.), *Contemporary neuropsychology and the legacy of Luria* (pp. 181–194). Lawrence Erlbaum Press.

Shultz, L. A. S., Pedersen, H. A., Roper, B. L., & Rey-Casserly, C. (2014). Supervision in neuropsychological assessment: A survey of training, practices, and perspectives of supervisors. *The Clinical Neuropsychologist, 28*(6), 907–925.

Stucky, K. J., Bush, S., & Donders, J. (2010). Providing effective supervision in clinical neuropsychology. *The Clinical Neuropsychologist, 24*(5), 737–758.

Tavris, C., & Aronson, E. (2008). *Mistakes were made (but not by me): Why we justify foolish beliefs, bad decisions, and hurtful acts*. Houghton Mifflin Harcourt.

Turnbull, O. H., Fotopoulou, A., & Solms, M. (2014). Anosognosia as motivated unawareness: The 'defence' hypothesis revisited. *Cortex, 61*, 18–29.

Turnbull, O. H., & Salas, C. E. (2017). Confabulation: Developing the 'emotion dysregulation' hypothesis. *Cortex, 87*, 52–61. https://doi.org/10.1016/j.cortex.2016.09.024

Walsh, K. (1992). Some gnomes worth knowing. *Clinical Neuropsychologist, 6*(2), 119–133. https://doi.org/10.1080/13854049208401849

1 We live or die by history

Rudi Coetzer

'Whoever wishes to foresee the future must consult the past'.

—Niccolo Machiavelli

1. Situation

After a few years in practice, clinicians start to develop confidence. A sense that all one could possibly encounter as a clinician must now have been seen. Every new patient starts to look just like all the others you have seen, with just minimal variation in the details of their histories. At this stage in one's development as a clinical neuropsychologist, it starts to feel as if you have assessed and followed so many patients with severe head trauma, heaps of people who have suffered stroke, many different types of brain infections, with the less common aetiologies sprinkled in between – like a never-ending conveyer belt of diverse pathologies, a wide range of onsets and presenting problems. By now, neuropsychologists may start to feel as if they had seen it all, listened to all the possible stories that patients bring to the consultation room, in all their various permutations.

At this stage, one of the main developmental tasks on the road to becoming a good clinical neuropsychologist includes (as in any profession) becoming more efficient, faster, but without losing accuracy. As Walsh (1985) so rightly pointed out, time is an expensive commodity in clinical practice. Speed is an important skill to hone, and even more so in large publicly funded hospitals, where the number of patients seen is huge. It is also the time where we begin to provide support to the next generation of clinicians, clinical trainees on placement. Gradually, it is not only your own cases you carry but also those of the colleagues you supervise. In effect, it is the beginning of the transition period to becoming 'an old hand'. Let's look at an example of how this situation might present itself to the clinical neuropsychologist.

2. Example

The remarkable thing about Ross was how ordinary he appeared. In the waiting room, I met a slightly built man with several faded tattoos all over his

DOI:10.4324/9781003300748-1

arms, neck and face. As we walked from the waiting room to my office, there seemed to be nothing obviously wrong with him – no hemiplegia, no bumping into objects, walking just fine. This first impression was confirmed when we sat down in my office to start the consultation. He was cooperative, nothing wrong with his speech, although he appeared ever so slightly reticent. No problem, he will soon warm to the situation, everybody is a bit anxious during a first hospital appointment, I thought. And nothing which years of experience and a good bedside manner cannot overcome. Although Ross made good eye contact, his expression of affect remained a bit limited in range, as well as intensity. Other than that, there was nothing particularly unusual.

When I asked Ross how I could help, he told me that he had been experiencing headaches, and from time to time, 'attacks'. I enquired about the nature and frequency of these, but he could not tell me much. 'I don't remember them, doctor' was his reply. I assumed that they were seizures, and remembered that in fact the referral did mention this. The headaches were bad from Ross' report, and he could describe these well – throbbing, accompanied by nausea and sensitivity to light. The only thing that helped was to 'sleep it off' in a dark room. Obviously, migraine. Right, I thought, now for the onset of these problems, and then all should be clear. Several other patients were waiting to be seen during the morning. Being slow with one patient does not at all help the many who also need to be attended to.

We got a little bit stuck with the next stage of the clinical assessment. Ross was slightly vague as to when his problems started, describing a more insidious onset. He said that about three years ago, while sitting in a bar, he was out of the blue suddenly assaulted, hit in the head by a local thug. He told me this rather casually. I was somewhat surprised to hear that he did not think much of it, as if it was an everyday event. He made a throwaway remark that 'they hit him hard', and that maybe it was a hammer rather than a fist. Ross said he got up from the floor and stumbled home. He remembers little, other than his wife being very cross when he arrived home 'drunk again'. He woke up (understandably) with a headache the next morning. Why was he not bothered by the assault? He said that it was just some thug he knew from the past and 'something that happened'. Ah, I thought, head trauma without extended loss of consciousness. Bet you he went to hospital within the next day or two, where all was revealed – most likely a slowly evolving sub-dural haemorrhage. Or perhaps, was he intoxicated, masking his confusion or post-traumatic amnesia?

Did he go to the hospital? He replied that he had not, nor did he see any doctor about it. Considering this new bit of information, to me it sounded like he was probably intoxicated already when he was assaulted, and that was why he was so vague? He would then have 'slept off the hangover' over the next few days after the injury. Things probably gradually improved, until the first seizure, perhaps a few weeks later. He would then have gone to hospital, and had all the clinical investigations required to confirm a diagnosis of post-traumatic seizures. I'd seen quite a few of these in the past. Just a bedside clinical assessment remaining now, and I would know if I needed to book him in for formal neuropsychological testing. Plus do a history, just for the sake of completeness. That's the way we were trained. Everybody was going to be seen on time for a change. And lunch was going to be early today.

On bedside cognitive testing, Ross' presentation wasn't especially complicated. He was right-handed, with one of his fingers (right hand) fairly heavily bandaged. He had several visible scars. He was neatly dressed, friendly and cooperative. He made good eye contact throughout the consultation, but I thought that his expression of affect was rather blunted. Indeed, he did not seem particularly bothered by anything. He remained vague, and perhaps at times a little bit parsimonious, in his answers to my questions. Was he avoiding something? Returning to the bedside examination, he was orientated to time, place and person. His speech was slightly monotone. As regards basic language functions, comprehension, repetition, naming, reading and writing were all grossly intact on bedside cognitive testing. He could list 17 animals in a minute. Apart from asking about orientation, I didn't assess his memory at this stage. And I was already starting to consider formally testing him.

A brief mental status examination revealed no reports of features consistent with a sustained depressed mood, but did say that he was feeling unhappy about some social problems he was experiencing. On closer questioning this transpired to be a problematic relationship with an ex-partner, but he was happily remarried now. Furthermore, he retained a good sense of future and certainly was not depressed, nor unduly anxious. He had no thoughts or plans to harm himself, or others. He did report that he sometimes struggled to fall asleep, without any early morning awakening. He said his appetite was good, and his weight remained constant at 65 kg. He thought his energy levels were good. And he denied experiencing any visual or auditory hallucinations. I deemed his thought processes to be entirely normal.

He provided me with a largely uncomplicated history. At this point of the assessment, I thought that he had settled and relaxed into the routine of the consultation, although he still appeared slightly slow and lacking in affective expression. He told me that he was born in a normal delivery. His developmental milestones were normal. He denied experiencing any health problems or hospital admissions as a child. In an increasingly 'average' account, he reported leaving school at the age of 18, with an academic performance that was about average compared to other kids in his school. But he had failed a year, due to becoming friendly with the 'wrong crowd'. He told me that after he completed his schooling, he 'drifted' for about 5 years, doing informal work here and there, and became involved in petty crime. During this period, he had some contact with the police and the criminal justice system, but denied ever serving a prison sentence. About 4 years later, he got a job as a packer at a small factory, and his life became much more settled. This is where he was working when he was assaulted.

Continuing with the uneventful history, there were no previous significant head injuries, loss of consciousness, admissions to hospital for psychiatric treatment, illnesses of note or other medical problems. He had been injured while playing rugby when he was younger, and once required attendance at the emergency department for a fractured collar bone. But he was on no medication. There was some history of potential substance misuse in the past, but he did not provide much detail. He only noted, with a wry smile, that all his friends smoked cannabis. Both Ross' parents were still alive, and there was no family history of note. As regards the collateral information available to me at the time, there were some suggestions from his co-workers in the factory that there had been changes in his behaviour and personality since his head injury. Apparently he had become lacking in social judgement, a bit more irritable and impulsive – but nothing especially notable.

And that was that. It all felt very much like the usual routine while seeing new patients in a busy clinic. The presentation and history appeared to fit quite well with a suspected head injury (traumatic brain injury) of some sort, with subtle psychological changes, headaches and seizures. As regards hypotheses, the cognitive impairments were then likely to also be subtle on testing, and might even possibly be masked by a reasonable level of pre-morbid schooling and intellectual ability, as was thought to be the case in Ross' situation. Indeed, this would not be an unusual presentation at all. Accordingly, an appointment for formal neuropsychological assessment was arranged, and he went on his way. I completed my clinic, and several more, before I saw Ross again. In the meantime, my mind was possibly elsewhere, as I was about to move house after accepting a new job in another city. I was on 'autopilot', while dealing with all the complexities involving the move.

Eventually Ross' follow-up appointment day came, and a quick look at my last few sentences in the notes reminded me that the plan was to test him. This would have been a rather standard approach, where bedside clinical examination revealed very little of note. Significant or obvious bedside findings do not require formal neuropsychological testing (Lezak et al., 2012). However, when there are subtle problems on bedside testing, formal testing is almost inevitably indicated. Unsurprisingly, Ross presented in the same manner as when I initially saw him a couple of weeks earlier. I duly completed a full neuropsychological testing, and scored everything up later that day. When I looked a bit more closely at the numbers, I was surprised. It was not what I expected. I checked my calculation of the percentiles, as I thought that the results were interesting. Or perhaps one shouldn't use 'results' in the plural? There was one interesting, isolated, result.

Ross had a completely normal, average set of percentiles in his test performance profile, except an obvious, gross impairment on one, and only one, test: *The Tower of Hanoi*. A performance quite obviously impaired, where he could only solve problems up to the three rings, and seven moves, level. Why was this clear failure on one test only? That's odd, I thought. Quite some head injury to result in such a specific, isolated impairment. But at least his impairment was on a (supposed) test of executive control function. Dysexecutive impairment is, of course, a hallmark cognitive impairment following traumatic brain injury (perhaps with new learning and slow information processing). Maybe then it was a focal injury. Focal? Did I miss something? Ross didn't lose consciousness at all.

Mercifully, before too long, a plausible answer came to me. Ross described experiencing seizures. All the data were now pointing to something more focal than contusions or diffuse axonal injury, following 'run of the mill' head trauma. In fact, now that I thought about it again, Ross reminded me of the few focal traumatic brain injuries I have seen over the past few years. In these cases, usually there was the presence of what was clearly a severe injury, including then a circumscribed depressed skull fracture, after being hit with for example a metal bar. And I reminded myself that Ross did mention something about a hammer, didn't he? Or was that a reference to the force of the fist hitting him? I was still not entirely convinced that my diagnostic formulation was correct, but at least it was plausible. And I had many other patients to see.

The fact that Ross had such a specific impairment continued to bother me. I decided to have another, closer, look at the rather cryptic referral. Once I read over it again, I was none the wiser. There was only one remaining option now to resolve the puzzle. I decided to take the long-walk upstairs to neurology to ask the consultant neurologist who made the referral. Would he mind showing me the CT or MRI films, to talk me through the findings on neuro-imaging? Particularly, it is in view of the odd neuropsychological assessment. The consultant looked pleased when he saw me, and asked his standard question, with a glint in his eye. What did I think of Ross' 'memory loss'? Comically, for this consultant, *every* type of cognitive impairment in clinical neuropsychology equalled 'memory loss'. I explained that he had no memory problems, but a rather circumscribed and significant impairment of executive function. Would it be possible for him to show me the neuro-imaging? The consultant beamed as he pulled out the CT film to show me. What on earth is he up to?

I always felt uneasy when he had *that* smile. . . . But everything was going to be OK, I thought. My consultant colleague was just, well . . . eccentric. He was probably first going to tell me to present the case, predict where the lesion(s) is, and then show me what was actually found. Just to remind me of the usual limitations in localising from neuropsychological test findings alone, without the benefit of neuro-imaging. It is a truism which of course I already knew. But it was his usual teaching routine. So I formulated the case in my mind, ready to present. It's a very useful skill to be able to present cases without the benefit of the file, as I was taught years ago. One should know your cases well enough to be able to do this. But while I was thinking, there is an interruption to my train of thoughts. Instead of asking me to present, he started to very briefly tell me the history I needed to make sense of the presentation. As he reported this, I gradually became aware of a vague sense of physical discomfort. It was quite hot here in the neurology ward. Do they not realise that it is summer and there is no need for extra heating? The temperature increased as the source of my unease started to reveal itself.

Initially, the consultant outlined essentially the same history I elicited from Ross. He was assaulted and hit to the head. And yes, there was no extended loss of consciousness. And he did indeed go home on his own volition. Yes, it is true that he never consulted a doctor. Yes, was I aware that he had seizures, I did ask? So, the consultant continued, did I ask Ross *exactly* what happened when he was assaulted? Come on, he had a head injury, I think. There was nothing else to ask? Every second patient we see is hit on the head. The consultant smiled. Actually, Ross was stabbed in the head. Well OK . . . it's no big deal, surely it's still the blow, the transfer of force, rather than a knife or whatever object was in the assailant's hand *per se*? It's the same acceleration/deceleration that causes any closed head injury, I ask the consultant. Not quite.

Did I remember that Ross' co-workers thought that his personality had changed? He used to be easy going and friendly. Now they said that he had become 'difficult', 'impulsive' and 'bothersome' – and always complaining of headaches. They *told* him that he should go to hospital. Indeed, it seems that Ross did go to a local community hospital, and said that he was sure that he must have cracked a bone in his head or face, because 'his head is sore', ever since he was in a fight, and was hit to the face and head. At triage a CT head with bone studies was requested. Whoever triaged Ross probably thought that he might have an old orbital, cheekbone or other facial fracture, and wanted to exclude this. They were probably unaware that his difficulties started several months ago, unsurprising given that he had up to that point not come to *any* healthcare professional's attention. However, the consultant was not sure of the exact circumstances surrounding their reasoning. At this stage I felt that our conversation was becoming a bit dull, and I just wished he would show me the CT film. He did. And there, unmissable, in the right frontal lobe sat, embedded, a broken off blade from the front of a knife. It literally took my breath away.

3. Errors

The missing piece (again literally) in Ross' assessment and integration had been a lack of focus on the most important part of the history. There had been lots of time on presenting complaints, bedside testing, formal testing and collateral information. But not enough focus on the exact circumstances surrounding sustaining his injury. It is not that I took a 'bad' history. In fact, it was rather comprehensive, including most of what would be needed during a first assessment of a new patient. The problem was not realising where in the history it was necessary to 'drill down' much deeper and to invest less time on (say) the developmental milestones, and more on requesting the full hospital records. All of the problems stemmed from that episode. Ross was vague about that episode, as one might expect from a man with a bit of knife still embedded in his frontal lobe. But I accepted Ross' vagueness. Not all parts of the history are equally important, and yet I allowed myself to gloss over what any sensible clinician would know as the most critical part. And so, amidst the distraction and ambiguity, I made a classic error.

Sometimes we, as clinical neuropsychologists, can jump to conclusions much too soon. A comprehensive pre-morbid history should be documented, but not at the cost of making sure of every *relevant* detail of the recent history. Those aspects must be explored in sufficient detail. Too much diagnostic confidence, too early in the assessment process, can come back to haunt you. In a sense, Ross' case was 'too easy', perfectly hiding the unexpected behind the many times encountered.

4. Reflection

Everyone notes the importance of practitioners having good clinical assessment skills. Naturally this includes the skill (and patience) to always take a thorough history and to never take short cuts, and never assume anything beforehand. If ever there were a clinical insurance policy, this is it. A patient's background information, or history, provides the context from within which to interpret the clinical findings. While having access to these contextual data of course does not guarantee *complete* accuracy, it can reduce the risk of errors. And, as we all know, blind analysis of neuropsychological test findings, without the relevant background information, is manifestly insufficient for complex clinical decision making (Lezak et al., 2012).

Perhaps there are other issues to consider as well. After a few years of working as a clinical neuropsychologist, every case starts to, as they say, 'merge into one'? However, that does not explain what went wrong in the assessment of Ross. There were distracters acting as red herrings. First, most patients we see look physically fine, as if there is nothing obviously wrong with them. Their neuropathology is invisible to us. We need an appropriate neuro-radiological investigation to look inside the skull. And even then, findings may be 'normal' – but more about that in a later chapter. Second, many, if not all, of the patients we proceed to formally test have *some* form of cognitive impairment. Furthermore, they often have cognitive impairment across more than one neuropsychological domain.

In a sea of what is mostly routine practice in everyday clinical neuropsychology work, it is exactly this, the 'ordinary', that tests us, and that eventually catches us out. Ross did indeed look very ordinary. But it is not what patients *look* like which helps us to correctly identify what is wrong. Presenting complaints are crucial, as is reading the clinical file, doing a collateral interview and looking at neuro-imaging. But ultimately, it is a patient's *history* that is critical. I am always reminded of a phrase cited by Walsh (one of his 'gnomes', though he borrowed it from Hampton et al., 1975) that 'Extra time spent on the history is likely to be more profitable than extra time spent on the examination' (Walsh, 1992, p. 123). How we reconstruct that history, without assuming anything, provides the unique 'fingerprint' that can colour the often-similar clinical presentation of a neuropathology. It is here where we can find the subtle clues, the context, that sheds light on the individual patient, and how they differ from the known communalities associated with their brain injury.

In essence, we 'live and die by history'. Which means that, in moderation, confidence is a good thing, in excess, it may be problematic.

A final question here is *why* clinicians jump to conclusions without collecting and examining the necessary evidence, *why* do we stop when more drilling is necessary. This is something not unusual, and newly qualified as well as experienced clinicians can make such mistake. We believe that there are two relevant factors here at play, a cognitive and an emotional one. The cognitive element is one that can be described as the tendency of human brains to predict what will happen based on what they already know (Bar 2011; Pally, 2007). In other words, humans, and clinical neuropsychologists are humans too, have the automatic predisposition to fill in the gaps in order to make sense. Filling in the gaps, by using our past experience, is a very efficient way to predict the future and guide our behaviour. As noted many years ago by Luria, brains do not perceive, they remember! (Luria, 1995 [1975]). The corollary of this idea is that story taking is a nearly impossible task. Or at least, a task that demands from us to temporarily resist – or inhibit – the natural tendency to *quickly* make sense. To extract as many pieces of the puzzle as we can before trying to put them all together, a theme we return to in the final chapter.

We also think that there is an emotional element at play when jumping into conclusions – an emotional factor that almost *compels* us to quickly make sense. When we make sense, and understand, it brings satisfying order and coherence. The relationship between order and well-being is an old idea in neuropsychological rehabilitation, proposed by Kurt Goldstein (1995 [1939]): 'In an ordered situation, responses appear to be constant, correct, adequate to the organism to which they belong . . . the individual himself experiences them with a feeling of smooth functioning, unconstraint, well-being . . . and satisfaction' (pp. 48–49). This adds a further complexity to our job as clinical neuropsychologists, for understanding a patient's case has emotional consequences for us. Famously, this conundrum is not exclusive of our peculiar discipline but applies to the psychotherapies as well.

In psychoanalytic theory, this problem has been theoretically addressed at some length. Some authors have proposed that clinicians should practice the ability to suspend Memory (how our perception is determined by what we know) and Desire (how our perception is determined by what we want) when attempting to understand the subjective experience of our patients. This 'ability' has been referred to as 'the Negative Capability of the therapist' (Bion, 1970), since it helps them not to 'saturate' the patient's narrative, and its meaning, with contents from their mind – thus, in order to listen the patient's own meaning. The negative capability would imply that we temporarily *withhold* our natural tendency to jump into conclusions, in order to see as many pieces as possible before making a diagnostic call. The training of such ability can be particularly relevant for young trainees, eager to prove that they 'understand', thus decreasing anxiety and confusion (an excess of Desire). It can also be equally relevant for the experienced clinician, who feels that they have already seen everything (an excess of Memory). We live or die by our ability to take a history, and, importantly, by the skill to withhold jumping to conclusions.

References

Bar, M. (2011). *Predictions in the Brain: Using Our Past to Generate a Future*. Oxford University Press: Oxford.

Bion, W. R. (1984 [1970]). *Attention and Interpretation*. Karnac Books: London.

Goldstein, K. (1995 [1939]). *The Organism: A Holistic Approach to Biology Derived From Pathological Data in Man*. The MIT Press: Cambridge.

Hampton, J. R., Harrison, M. J. G., Mitchell, J. R. A., Pritcbard, J. S., & Seymour, C. (1975). Relative contributions of history taking, physical examination, and laboratory investigation to diagnosis and management of medical out-patients. *British Medical Journal* 2: 486–489.

Lezak, M. D., Howieson, D. B., Bigler, E. D., & Tranel, D. (2012). *Neuropsychological Assessment* (5th ed.). Oxford University Press: New York.

Luria, A. (Luria, 1995 [1975]). *Sensación y Percepción*. Ediciones Martínez-Roca: Barcelona.

Pally, R. (2007). The predicting brain: Unconscious repetition, conscious reflection and therapeutic change. *The International Journal of Psychoanalysis* 88 (4): 861–881.

Walsh, K. (1992). Some gnomes worth knowing. *Clinical Neuropsychologist* 6 (2): 119–133. doi: 10.1080/13854049208401849.

Walsh, K. W. (1985). *Understanding Brain Damage. A Primer of Neuropsychological Evaluation*. Churchill Livingstone: Edinburgh.

2 The wrong amnesia

Oliver Turnbull

'When you have to make a choice and don't make it, that in itself is a choice'.
—William James

1. Situation

Humans have a wonderful habit of continuing down the paths which they've already started. The world puts something interesting out there, down a route that you've followed before, and people will sail down the well-trodden pathway, without a moment's consideration that they might have made a poor choice. There's a reason that, in the famous poem, Robert Frost's character is remarkable for choosing the unusual or exceptional route: the road 'less travelled'. The poem is (arguably) famous because the character is admirable in making an unusual choice.

Why do we stick to well-trodden paths? Partly because they are easy and familiar: you have the skills that you need, things seem fluent, familiar and safe. And also because of the dark side of realising that you're on the *wrong* path. That would be admitting that you made a mistake, that you were wrong. That would mean change, and uncertainty.

What then is the risk for the early career neuropsychologist? There may be something about a clinical presentation that suggests an obvious route of investigation – perhaps it is the patient's complaint, or the lesion visible on scan. You know how to investigate this one, and you start down the path. And it's a comfortable feeling. It's amazing how, with just a little confirmation bias, it's possible not to notice that you've gone awry. But once you are on the wrong path, it can be too late.

What should you have done instead? Perhaps stepped back, every now and then, to check your assumptions, and the state of your evidence? Does it all add up? And if it doesn't, can you be brave enough to check and see whether you were wrong? To try and disconfirm your hypothesis? Everyone talks about how science works by stress-testing your ideas through disconfirmation. But hardly anyone does this. Indeed, scientists are famously prone to confirmation bias too. There are reasons for why an Albert Einstein or a Marie Curie only comes along occasionally.

DOI:10.4324/9781003300748-2

The case here is, alas, one of those 'familiar route' errors – a safe, well-rehearsed path, which I followed as a naïve trainee. I won't make the same mistake twice.

2. Example

When he entered the room, it wasn't immediately obvious that David had a memory problem. In fact, David *himself* wasn't all that obvious, given that he seemed metaphorically hidden in the shadow of Mrs Merton, his mother. She was an energetic woman, whom one suspected had encountered a number of difficulties in her life, and had circumvented or bulldozed her way past almost all of them. Yes, she was a little early for the meeting, but she was always punctual, she told me. No, she wouldn't be happy to leave me to speak to David alone. It would be much easier if she explained things, because she understood them more clearly than he did. And it would save time – she was always good at saving time, she continued.

I took a deep breath, and then Mrs Merton was off again. Yes, things had been difficult since David had his car accident – almost three years ago now. He'd always been a lively, friendly child, she said. Normal milestones, did fine at school, doing all-right in a job at the supermarket, perhaps hung around with the wrong crowd, a little too much drinking on the weekend. And then the car accident, just near the off-ramp from the motorway – perhaps I'd seen it in the newspapers? It seemed as if she had been in the room for 10 minutes before either David or myself had had a chance to even open our mouths to speak.

Given that I was a trainee in my 20s, and Mrs Merton was a take-no-prisoners mother of 3 in her late 40s, I think I managed a valiant attempt at wresting some control over the meeting from her. If there was one thing I knew from my training, it was that I should establish the principal complaint, and take the history, from the *patient* first, and *then* the family. There were all sorts of things that patients might say (or indeed not say) that it was going to be good to hear from the patient first. So I directed the interview towards David. Did he agree with his mother's account of the history? Yes, that was a good summary. Including the accident? Again, he said that agreed with his mother. Indeed, it was becoming clear that it was perhaps *always* safer to simply agree with David's mother – probably on almost all topics. Just for the sake of a quiet life.

And so, what was his principal complaint – what was the main thing that was troubling him at the moment? His memory, he said. He was really forgetful. Yes, Mrs Merton chipped in, and launched into a summary, and a series of anecdotes: he didn't remember to do chores round the house, he forgot meetings with his friends, much less hospital appointments, didn't remember birthdays, didn't keep up with the news, he would sometimes forget what a word was, and she had to remind him. I was tempted to point out to her that her last example was really better classified as anomia than an example of recent memory impairment. But it didn't seem worth the trouble. I turned to David again. Did he agree that his mother was correct about the nature of the problem – that he forgot things that had happened in the last few minutes, hours and days? Yes. How bad was it? Bad, he said. He was always forgetting things. Absolutely, said Mrs Merton: So, so forgetful – memory like a sieve!

So far, so good, I thought. Amnesia – I was on to something. And so, to the history, to document the rest of the classic profile of amnesia. Could he remember things for a few seconds, like 'No ifs ands or buts'? He repeated it perfectly. When did his problems begin? After the accident. His memory had been pretty good before that. And so to retrograde: How was his memory from before the accident? Like every other closed head injury patient, he didn't remember the accident. What was the last thing he remembered from before the accident? Earlier that day. And after the accident? He wasn't sure. A little bit of to and fro with Mrs Merton and David established the details of that: perhaps a week or two before he had stopped being confused. But his memory had never returned to normal. And the memory for things well before the accident – weeks, months years? Just fine.

So, a nice tidy case for the morning. It had been a motor vehicle accident, with a fairly classic few hours of retrograde amnesia, and a few weeks of post-traumatic amnesia. Really quite a substantial post-traumatic amnesia, actually, which meant that he was expected to present with the usual range of executive impairments. Not that I'd noticed much of the dysexecutive presence in the interview, though David had seemed distractable, admittedly. He hadn't always seemed to pay attention to what his mother was saying, and his answers hadn't always got to the heart of the matter. However, as regards inhibition, he had been quiet, and socially appropriate. But perhaps he wasn't in the mood for being disinhibited with his mother in the room? I made a note to make sure that I tested him alone. That part of the testing should be easy: run him past a range of the usual executive measures and see what pops out. I knew enough from my training thus far not to make too many assumptions about *which* executive measure he might fail on, but he was entitled to failure, I might well see a few things emerge when he was out from under his mum's shadow.

The question now was *what* I might see when David was on his own with me. There was one part of the history that really didn't make sense: his current memory problems. Why did he have a memory impairment? He was 'So, so forgetful', apparently? Every trainee knows that so-called 'axial' amnesia, the severe memory impairment seen after lesions to the hippocampus and the like, doesn't usually follow from the sort of damage caused by acceleration-deceleration trauma. The stretching, tearing and micro-bleed lesions tended to happen primarily in the orbital frontal and anterior temporal lobes.

However, closed head injury could produce damage in unexpected places. I seemed to recall that the main cause was bleeds, again from stretched and torn arteries. And there was another cause of hippocampal damage after traumatic injury: the hypoxia that follows from vascular problems elsewhere in the body. I knew this because I'd heqrd about an amnesic patient a few weeks earlier, on a ward round. After a very serious heart attack, he'd been hypoxic, and I'd remembered that one part of the hippocampus (I'd forgotten the exact name) was especially vulnerable to reductions in oxygen supply. So perhaps David had something that had caused a lot of bleeding? I dug out the notes. Had there been any other injury as part of the car accident? Indeed there had. A fairly serious shoulder injury, now largely resolved, but it looked like a candidate for the bleed. Bingo. All I needed to do was document the severity of the memory impairment, and check whether he really was dysexecutive or not.

Having persuaded Mrs Merton to wait outside, the assessment proceeded smoothly. A measure of premorbid intelligence suggested that he would have been of average intelligence. But it became increasingly clear – as predicted – that his executive function wasn't matching that pre-morbid level. He wasn't doing too badly on some executive measures, but then again he was really failing on others. With lists of word by starting letter, he could find lots of words that began with S, but the list of 'legal' words (sun, sin, sign, simple, etc.) was scattered amongst rule violations: a few things starting with capital letters, such as people, products and places. So we had 'Sarah, Simon and Snickers'. And, as the test wore on, we had wasteful repetitions of sun and simple.

Perhaps David had forgotten the rules, so I reminded him about the people, products and places violations. Yes, he said, he remembered the rules, he said. But I'd told him to name as many things as possible, so he was just getting stuck in! Just the sort of excuse that our dysexecutive patients normally gave me. And we all make mistakes, he said. It would be interesting to see whether he had decent error-utilisation? Could he keep the rules in mind for when we tried the next letter? Of course he could, he said. And yet we soon had France and Philip sprinkled amongst free, friendly and famous. Things took a turn for the worse when we tried the letter A: he started to riff on asshole, ass-wiper and then ass-licker . . . all with a smile on his face. I was left wondering how to score the offending items, and indeed what his mother might have said had she been in the room. In addition, all of this was an interesting answer to my earlier query about how his disinhibition might be related to his mother's presence. Disinhibited he might be, but apparently not disinhibited enough to cross her. Doubtless based on a lot of life experience!

It was becoming increasingly obvious that he was a distractable, rather disinhibited young man. He did manage Trail Making Part A, with its joining of well-learned sequences. But he needed a second explanation of how the more complicated Part B worked. And then he really took his time on it – it was hard to tell whether he was bored, or struggling. The other difficult moment was in the Wisconsin, which started badly, as he failed to grasp the instructions. Once we were up and running, he managed (through luck or judgement) to hit upon 'colour' as the concept. But he just couldn't manage the first shift *from* colour to form. After what turned out to be one too many of my 'No' responses to his perseveration in colour-sort choices, he gave a little punch to the desk, then shot me a look that said 'One step further and I'll deck you, mate!'. He did nothing, fortunately, but both of us knew that we'd crossed a line, and I'd seen how much volatility there was behind that passive and distractable façade. I terminated the test, and we took a break.

So, half of the job was done. All I lacked were some memory tests. I was especially interested in measures of recent memory, which were at the heart of any axial amnesia. And I'd be wanting to do some non-verbals as well as verbals. I tried the Story Recall. He managed about half of it, wandering off on to an anecdote about his friend on a fishing boat, and not recalling much more, even when I brought him back on track. One more verbal memory test, again poor: after three attempts, he was hopeless with the difficult paired associates, even when I asked him to guess – next, to something visual. He was bad, but not terrible, in drawing from immediate memory. I tried the Rey Figure. Not the smartest copy I'd ever seen, and after a delay a pretty shoddy recall – mostly the main architecture, and no real detail. At least we were making progress. I just needed to confirm that his immediate memory was intact. He needed a few re-tries on forwards Digit Span, but got to 6. His backwards Digits were really suspect, at 3, but I knew to attribute that to his executive impairment. So, I was happy to tick him off as an axial amnesic too. All I needed to do was write the report, and try to avoid looking too smug when I presented the findings on pathology expertly identified in not one but two brain regions.

3. Error

Presenting the findings to my supervisor was a game of two halves. First is the history of closed head injury, and the associated executive impairments. Nothing exciting here, but I was getting some credit for noting the disinhibition, and mentioning the likely orbito-frontal cause of the problem. In retrospect, perhaps I should have re-interpreted the raised eyebrow when I mentioned axial amnesia. When I mentioned it a second time the raised eyebrow became a 'Really?'. But I was allowed to run all the way through my presentation before the questioning began. In retrospect, I should have realised that I was digging myself into a hole on the amnesia issue, but perhaps a part of me thought that I could bluster it out – like Mrs Merton, if I said things with enough confidence, the world might agree with me.

Now it was the turn of the questions. How did I know it was an axial amnesia? It was because of the poor memory performance on the Wechsler. It seemed obvious. And it was a recent memory impairment in both the visual and verbal domains? Yes, David had done quite badly on *lots* of the recent memory subtests. And doing badly *both* on the visual and verbal measures meant that . . . ? It meant that the lesion must be bilateral, I replied? By now I suspected that this was going to end badly. And the pathology that caused the bilateral hippocampal lesions was going to be . . . ? Some sort of hypoxic damage, I'd imagined. And caused by the blood loss from the peripheral injury. A long pause from my supervisor before the next question. Not a good sign. So, this memory impairment, could there be any other cause . . . anything other than an axial amnesia? I paused and tried to think, but my mind was blank. Er, no, I said. He'd done badly on all the measures of recent memory on the Wechsler – it 'had' to be an axial amnesia?

4. Reflection

So, to return to the 'pathway' analogy that opened the chapter, what was the wrong path that I'd taken, and why had I stayed on it? The start of the problem was failing to listen to the complaint properly. First, I had to listen 'like a neuropsychologist', not like someone taking dictation. Mrs Merton had told me that David had a memory impairment, and I was right to have believed her. But to listen like a clinician is to think of the many ways that a system can fail. Certainly, the heart of memory is the episodic systems of the Papez circuit – where lesion produces the classic axial amnesia. But there are many other reasons for memory to fail: like not concentrating on the material, not organising the material, and not being motivated to remember. Perhaps I could have listened to Mrs Merton differently? That included better listening to her narrative? That David 'didn't remember to do chores round the house, forgot meetings with his friends, didn't remember birthdays', and so on. Are those the errors made in axial amnesia? Certainly. Can those errors be produced for other reasons? Absolutely.

On reflection, I could have listened more effectively, and not become stuck wandering down the Papez path. Second, once I was *on* the path, I could have considered and weighed up whether that line of argument was appropriate? Was David *really* behaving like an axial amnesic? Part of the problem was that, so early in my career, I hadn't actually seen an axial amnesic. But even that early on my career, I should have been able to see that he *wasn't* incapable of remembering, if the material was something he cared about? Then I could have walked away, and reconsidered the case in the round. But that would have been a brave, clinically sophisticated, move – but I was too inexperienced. So, what do we know about memory, and the many ways that the system can fail?

Like all complex psychological skills, memory requires the engagement of a number of distinct processes. Many textbooks focus on the core abilities – usually classified as encoding, storage and retrieval: how memories are laid down, developed into well-established traces, and how can they be retrieved. Almost 150 years of memory research has taught us a great deal about these abilities – such as the well-known primacy and recency effects. This line of enquiry has also shown us very clearly that rehearsal and 'depth' of processing seem central to the laying down of a secure memory trace. We remember things much more effectively when it fits with our general understanding of the world, as a jigsaw piece within our existing semantic network. It's easier to remember the orderly sequence of '11, 13, 15, 17', rather than the incoherent jumble of '24, 83, 41, 13'. Memories are also better remembered when they are rehearsed – in the way that we re-recalled our first kiss a lot (as it was emotion-laden and unique), but we perhaps didn't recall out the thousandth kiss with our spouse (as things become less novel and exciting). So, we can be rather good at recalling material that is meaningful and well rehearsed.

The biological basis by which these sorts of memories are stored is well understood too. They do indeed involve the axial structures that I was so interested in with David. A classic axial amnesia would follow from any bilateral lesion to the hippocampus, para-hippocampal gyrus, fornix, mammillary bodies, mammilo-thalamic tract or anterior thalamic nucleus. We know that these brain systems do not themselves *hold* the recent memories, but they are central to the ability to lay such memories down, to create the connections that form an episode, and lesions to them produce classic, dense amnesias – which is why the textbooks spend most of their time on those core memory processes.

However, the implementation of all complex psychological skills is just that – complex. No neuropsychologist clarifies this as Luria does, and the later chapters of his classic text *The Working Brain* (1973) outline, step by step, the many processes, or components as Luria liked to described them, that underpin abilities such as problem-solving, action, language and memory. In each case, he outlines the diverse range of skills that contribute to even relatively simple mental achievements. Luria (1966) has some very clear comments on Kurt Goldstein's seminal paper 'The Symptom, its origin and significance' (1926):

> The symptom cannot be regarded as an immediate expression of the damaged function: it has to be analysed, and only an analysis of the basic disturbance which has to be singled out can show its real essence; this basic disturbance can solve the riddle of the whole syndrome – and only when it becomes clear is the clinical analysis of the patient over.
>
> (p. 312)

In my opinion, Luria's best example in *The Working Brain* is the chapter on problem-solving, where he constantly emphasises how important it is that we first *realise* that there is a problem to solve. Most authors dash into the fun parts of problem-solving: how does the agent choose between the competing potential solutions to a problem – so that the reader is immediately thinking about decision heuristics and supervisory attentional systems. Not Luria. As he points out, not realising that there *is* a problem to solve is a key impairment for many patients with frontal lesions.

Thus, it is with memory. It is true that axial brain systems are at the heart of successfully encoding the recent memory. But we must not forget the various *non*-memory components that need to operate successfully in order for encoding to succeed. They are the very skills that allow for those core elements of depth of processing and rehearsal. Skills such as organising the material to make it more meaningful, sustaining attention while this takes place, of realising that something is of sufficient importance to merit attempts at rehearsal, and then maintaining focus – and avoiding distraction – for this to be achieved. These are not skills mediated by axial brain systems like the hippocampus and the mammillary bodies. Rather they are *executive* skills – of the management and regulation of basic cognitive systems. And they are run in large part by the frontal lobes, and their connections.

So, did David have damage to two entirely independent brain regions: the frontal lobes *and* the hippocampus? That was possible, of course. But it wasn't the solution suggested by Occam's razor: *one* site of injury, disruption to *one* psychological process, would surely be a more elegant solution. However, in the best detective novels, one needs a key piece of evidence that will separate the two suspects. I was claiming that David had impairment to executive function and core recent memory systems. My supervisor was claiming that the impairment to recent memory systems was secondary to executive dysfunction. Was there a way to separate them out?

It was no fun having my supervisor lecture me about jumping to conclusions in relation to the amnesia. I didn't enjoy the fact that the phenomenon already had a label ('Frontal', or executive amnesia), which I appear to have heard about as a graduate student, but had conveniently forgotten (I couldn't help but think that I'd probably forgotten because I hadn't deployed enough depth of processing, or rehearsal . . .). And I particularly didn't enjoy the mention of Occam's razor. In my undergraduate years I'd had many an argument with 'less-rational' souls who seemed to believe in conspiracy theories, spoon-bending and astrology. I'd thrown the Occam's razor jibe at every one of them, and it was no fun having the argument applying to me for once. The only bright side to the difficult conversation was that my supervisor had produced a possible answer to the dilemma – a way that we *could* establish whether the recent memory impairment was secondary to the executive problems.

We waited for the next meeting with David and Mrs Merton, and then ensured that Mrs Merton wasn't in the room. It was only going to take a few minutes to do what we needed to do. My supervisor and I chatted to David for a few minutes, and asked him a few more questions. Not from dull psychological tests in which he had no interest, but for things that were likely to have meaning in his life, things which he was likely to want to rehearse. Was he a fan of sport? Football. Huge. Always had been. How had his team done on the weekend? His eyes lit up. Fantastic game, he said. Then launched into an account of the achievements of centre-forward x, and the failings of goal-keeper y. My supervisor shot a glance at me, as if to say 'And this is an amnesic?'. And how had the national team done in the World cup last month? Terrible, he said. If only that idiot of a coach (whom he named) had selected more players from his (David's) team – the best team, obviously – it wouldn't have been that fiasco against Portugal. Indeed. How many amnesics remember the details of things that happened last month – unless they really cared about the fiasco against Portugal, and had perhaps spent time going over the details of the match with their friends. Occam's razor was looking pretty sharp.

The only test that we wanted to do wasn't even standardised. My supervisor took off his watch, took out a pen, his wallet and dragged a stapler across the office desk. Then went through each of the four objects, over and over again – focusing on details, making jokes about them, engaging David in a discussion about them, and every now and then hiding one or two and asking where they were hidden. The pen was silver, getting a bit old and tarnished, could you see? But perhaps we won't throw it out yet – but *let's hide it behind the bin*? And the wallet – black, lots of University cards, not many credit cards, or much cash, eh? Don't pay us very much at the University these days. *We'll hide that behind the curtain.* Now where was that pen? What colour was it again? Here it is. Silver. Bit crappy at the end and so on. Five minutes of enforced attention for David. Simple ideas, easy associations. Lots of repetition. The reader already knows what happened when we asked him, 10 minutes later, what were the objects and where they were hidden. The part that shocked me the most was when I saw David again a few weeks later, in the same office. Unprompted, he had a few observations, almost as if he was showing off. Did that bloke ever throw away that old silver pen, he said? The one he hid behind the bin? And I suppose there's no point in looking behind the curtain to see whether the wallet's still there? Hardly anything in it anyway. Some amnesia.

References

Goldstein, K. (1926). Das Symptom, seine Entstehung und Bedeutung für unsere Auffassung vom Bau und von der Funktion des Nervensystems. *Archiv für Psychiatrie und Nervenkrankheiten*, 76(1), 84–108.

Luria, A. R. (1966). Kurt Goldstein and neuropsychology. *Neuropsychologia*, 4, 311–313.

Luria, A. R. (1973). *The working brain*. London: Penguin Books.

3   No such thing as a neuropsychological test

Oliver Turnbull

'In a very real sense there is virtually no such thing as a neuropsychological test'.
'Only the method of drawing inferences about tests is neuropsychological'.

—Kevin Walsh (1992) *Some gnomes worth knowing*

1. Situation

Training in any discipline, including neuropsychology, is a journey towards competence, towards expertise and fluency. All of which are wonderful things, linked as they are to feelings of well-being, control and confidence. However, expertise also brings a challenge, whenever a newly minted expert is faced with the unknown, and is therefore faced with a choice. On the one hand, this growing sense of expertise and fluency can lead to over-confidence – the impression that knowing *many* things means that one knows *every*thing. The alternative path, the developmental achievement, is the more difficult route to take, and requires that you realise when you are *out* of your comfort zone. And what should we do when we are in this difficult state? In theory, it should be clear what to do in that moment: consider alternative accounts; return to fundamentals; seek help. . . . Or at very least pause and take a deep breath.

We ask this of our patients all the time in therapeutic settings. You have a problem managing your anger after your brain injury? We can help you, by getting you to realise when you have *low* levels of anger. When you feel irritable, or frustrated, then evaluate whether you might be in a setting that could escalate to full blown anger, or even rage? Are you at risk of getting too frustrated? Then (because good therapy always benefits from a little analogy) you are like a traffic light that has turned from green to orange. Perhaps the patient might count to ten, or go and talk to someone else, or leave the room? Anything to avoid moving from orange to red.

Perhaps, as clinicians, we should heed our own advice? Whenever we are out of our comfort zone, whenever we feel that we have over-extended our expertise, then we should rate ourselves as green-to-orange and consider alternative accounts; return to fundamentals; or seek help. It's a difficult lesson to learn, as tricky for clinicians as it is for patients. But, potentially, it's a really valuable lesson.

DOI:10.4324/9781003300748-3

This case is an example where anyone sensible might have advised me to behave like someone outside of their comfort zone. In fact, I was literally entering a new 'zone' of the hospital, dealing with a different sort of patient, where my hard-won expertise in neuroanatomy and neuropathology was going to be of very little use. More importantly, there was going to be an entirely *different* set of expertise, in domains as diverse as social history and psychopharmacology, of which I knew worryingly little. Perhaps the most important aspect of expertise is knowing when you *don't* have it. When you have left your home turf – physically or metaphorically – then that's the time to ask the locals or read some unfamiliar textbooks. Alas, I did neither.

2. Example

I had never seen a patient like Peter before. I'd seen lots of patients, of course – I wasn't that new a trainee. But, as I took the history, it was progressively dawning on me that Peter was different from *every* one of them. The main difference was that the lives of the other patients had been dramatically transformed, from a premorbid existence that had apparently been quite normal. Of course, there was some variation by social class or gender. But they were all people whose conventional lives had suddenly been transformed by being unable to move part of their body, or speak fluently, or remember what happened yesterday. They came with loving-if-distressed family, and with careers of variable success. But they were all variations of conventional past lives, now shattered. I hadn't realised it before I met Peter, but the history of my adult neurology patients always had a clear sense of *before* (before the stroke, before the tumour) and *after*.

Peter was nothing of this. He didn't come with a spouse, children – nor any significant other that he mentioned positively. And, even though he was in his 40s, he didn't dress much like my 40-something neurology patients. He was all long hair and stubble, colourful shirts and a festival of wrist-bands. A very avant-garde look, had it been brought off with less of a sense that not much had been washed, ironed or combed in quite a while. Taking the history wasn't easy either: because there was so *much* of it. The difficult early family relationships, with a hint of physical abuse; the moves to different homes and schools; the poor school performance and early departure from education; the alcohol and some drugs; some vague attempts at work, combined with scraping by on social support; and a series of minor get-rich-quick schemes with so-called friends, which never quite seemed to work out. The longer I listened, the less it conformed to the 'I was normal and happy until my stroke/accident' model – the one that I was so used to.

The narrative was so different because today I'd strayed outside the Neurology ward and was on my first solo visit to Psychiatry. I knew the conceptual difference between the disciplines very well, of course. There had been enough formal teaching over the years to make that clear. But, based on a sample of one, I was coming to the conclusion that the differences appeared to start long before the onset of the 'official' symptoms, and the referral to the relevant professional. We finally *did* get to the 'initial' (if that was the phrase) onset of Peter's symptoms. This was in the late teenage years, seemingly coinciding with one or other of the alcohol and drug phases, sandwiched between episodes of chaotic family life.[1] But even that suggested date of onset wasn't adding much value. It was as if there wasn't a *pre*-morbid for Peter – but rather a series of warm-up acts.

Still, it wasn't my job to offer a psychiatric opinion. That was already well documented, in a file far thicker than the ones I was used to in Neurology. One of several psychiatrists seemed to think that 'schizophrenia' might be the best label. Or perhaps schizo-affective disorder? Indeed, to add to my growing lack of certainty, scattered through the notes there were other alternative or additional suggestions from the DSM. Anxiety and depression were common mentions, as well as ADHD? There was even one suggestion of OCD. Reading the notes had left me somewhere between co-morbidity, and people throwing darts at a board. I was starting to feel nostalgic for the clarity of signs and symptoms down the corridor in Neurology.

So, what was my job? Apparently, my job is to offer an opinion on a *neurological* disorder in our psychiatric patient. We had a referral, from what turned out to be a young and enthusiastic Registrar in Psychiatry, who had wondered whether the patient had a neurological disorder of one type or another. Peter had changed over the last few months, so she reported. The staff said that he was quieter at times, but at times more agitated, troubling the nurses in his unit, and occasionally turning on them in frustration. What could change in the course of adult schizophrenia, so the argument ran? So perhaps Peter had a novel onset disorder – hence the referral to Neurology. One of our young and enthusiastic neurologists had duly appeared, shone a light into some pupils, scraped the soles of feet and had announced nothing of neurological note. The pair of Registrars were then mulling up whether or not to spend the money on a scan. But, then as now, such procedures can be an expensive and imprecise tool of investigation, and neuropsychology seemed like another way in. And that was how I came to meet Peter, who was currently expanding my horizons, not only about *how* to take a history but even about what a history consisted *of*.

The case presented all sorts of problem-solving challenges that I'd never really grappled with before. First, Peter already *had* a medical diagnosis, a psychiatric one, that it seemed that it was primarily my job to *ignore*? Or at very least, I should try to work around it? So, when he started discussing his homegrown conspiracy theory, about the chemicals which the government was introducing into the water . . . then that probably was more of a psychiatric than a neuropsychological issue. Indeed, he told me, secretively, that he boiled and purified everything he drank.

However, I was more interested in what appeared to be a memory failure or two. For example, he produced a little anecdote about his psychiatrist's dress sense—early on in the interview, and then repeated the story to me an hour later. Had he forgotten that he'd told me? If these sorts of slips were a memory impairment, then that seemed much more interesting to a neuropsychologist than a conspiracy theory in a patient with a known psychiatric disorder. In retrospect, I realised that his repetition of significant themes across the interview may have been driven more by his obsessive interests than by memory impairment. The issue of government interference in the water supply, and his boiling and purifying, came up a second time too, and then much later a third. This was probably because he was obsessionally tied to the issue – after all, it was life-threatening to him. But, with hindsight, I didn't see the obsessional thinking. All I saw was a patient repeating an anecdote, which was simply confirmation of my 'it's a memory impairment' theory.

The other problem that I was faced with was 'where' to look. With time, I would come to really appreciate the referral letters that specified a particular issue: 'Could Mr Smith return to work after his right middle cerebral artery stroke?', 'Why was Mrs Jones not making any progress with her physiotherapists after her anterior communicating artery aneurysm?' and 'Was Mrs Thomas "entitled" to her amnesia, after her right posterior cerebral artery stroke?' These were beautifully constrained as a task: We had known pathology, we had site of lesion. This 'entitled' the patient, or narrowed the field down, to a short list of perhaps half a dozen neuropsychological disorders. I could quickly check that the requisite 'other' bits of the mind/brain were intact and then use the history, and some or other test, to measure the severity of the entitled deficits. Thus: function x was indeed impaired and was modest/severe/profound in its magnitude. First phase was done.

These findings then led back to the referral letter, which had so concisely asked why the patient wouldn't, or couldn't, do something in everyday life, or in therapy? Thus, I could use my neuropsychological knowledge to establish a possible answer all of those earlier questions: Mr Smith couldn't yet return to work after his right middle cerebral artery stroke, because he had mild hemispatial neglect, and I didn't want to be on the road near the lorry he'd be driving. Mrs Jones might not be making progress with her physiotherapists, not only because she had some sensory impairment in her lower limbs but also because she was adynamic, and therefore disengaged with therapy. Mrs Thomas was indeed 'entitled' to her amnesia, not least because she had a unilateral hippocampal lesion but also because she was ambidextrous, so she might well have anomalous cerebral dominance, and her right hippocampus might be very important, even for verbal memory. All of this was tidy, orderly neuropsychology, and I was very much enjoying being a tidy, orderly neuropsychologist.

3. Error

But Peter's referral was nothing like that of the neurological patients. There was no established pathology, and no likely lesion site – only a vague date of onset of 'a few months ago', and a short list of similarly vague symptoms relating to passivity, contrasting with the agitation and aggression. The start date and evolution suggested any number of pathologies, including brain tumour, or some sort of toxic or metabolic disorder, perhaps something degenerative . . . none of which seemed to have been formally excluded in the notes? Except that the basics of a neurological examination had turned up nothing of note, and I knew enough to know that normal pupils, optic fundii and reflexes allowed me to exclude a fair few things.

Later in my clinical career, I would undoubtedly have gone back to either the psychiatrist or the neurologist or both, and had a much clearer discussion about the likely (or even the possible) pathologies and lesion site. However, I was young, and I'd received a referral letter in a busy and fast-paced hospital. So, I blundered on with the only path that seemed sensible at the time, some sort of 'global' assessment. That was the start of the error: I was out of my depth, over-extended from my comfort zone.

How could I know this? Not least because I wasn't trying to answer a tightly framed hypothesis. The rest of my training had all been about a link between phenomena at different levels: a disorder of *function* x, which was run by *brain region* y, and had been disrupted by *disease process* z. I certainly did not have those three lined up here, and that should have rung alarm bells. What I *should* have done was pause, take a deep breath, then start to become better informed about psychiatric disorders, and reconsider the fundamentals. And, perhaps most importantly, this would have been a very good time to have sought help? Instead, I had chosen to start a journey, but I didn't have a properly chosen destination.

To make things even worse, Peter also denied that he had any of the problems listed in the letter. Sure, he felt tired, he said. Always had, more or less. And his memory wasn't too good either, he reported. He wondered whether that had something to do with the water . . . and we were back in the land of conspiracy theories! It was becoming clear that discussions were going to take us to unproductive places. Instead, I tried to work my way round the brain from first principles. A key element of my education in assessment was that I could skim over broad psychological functions, by giving high-level complex tasks. If the patient performed well, then I could have some confidence that the fundamentals were sound. So, if the patient could draw and recall the Rey Figure, then a range of basic visuo-spatial and visuo-motor abilities were probably fine, as well as spatial memory and perhaps executive function. Again, if the patient could fluently describe the Cookie Theft picture, then I wouldn't have much worry about object recognition, and some of the other visuo-spatial abilities, and expressive language, and again executive function . . . and so on. In this way, I worked my way round Peter's brain, with a few of these high-level measures, knowing that if he failed any of them, then I could investigate them in more detail later.

This seemingly basic approach was, alas, complicated in Peter's case: not least because so much of his neuropsychological performance was contaminated by the psychiatric features. His language was fine, except that the running tap in the Cookie Theft picture opened the conspiracy theory argument yet again! However, by and large, he was doing fine: no visuo-spatial or visuo-motor disabilities, no obvious language or spatial memory impairment. However, his performances were both unimpressive and also rather variable. His copy of the Rey Figure was a bit sloppy and disorganised, and as a consequence his recall wasn't catastrophic, but it was clearly poor. A good marker for executive impairment, I remembered. And his Cookie Theft description had all the fundamental objects in the scene: a mother dries dishes, a sink is over-flowing, children climb a chair to get cookies. But the story lacked the coherent narrative that might come from a more abstract interpretation: that the *reason* for the overflowing sink was the distracted mother, and her distraction *also* explained why the children were able to engage in cookie theft – again, another nod towards executive impairment.

At last I felt like a neuropsychologist: this was a problem I could handle! All I needed were some more measures of executive function – simple in theory. But, in reality, it took several hours over the rest of the day, because Peter was forever getting bored, or wanting to talk about the water supply, or taking a break for what seemed like a very serious nicotine habit. But by close of play I had more clarity. On some measures of executive function, he did well, on others less so. I couldn't see a pattern, but luckily, I wasn't floored by the variation. Everything I knew about executive function told me that it produced variable test performance: depending on the patient's fluctuating levels of concentration and motivation.

I even remembered to try some interventions to work *around* the concentration difficulty. On the memory tests, Peter did badly on Paired Associate Learning, forgetting pairs like cabbage-pen. The beginner's error, I remembered, was to assume that poor performance on this memory test automatically meant a memory impairment. So, I re-administered it, this time acting as an external source of executive function and building a mnemonic for him. The cabbage-pen link was easy to remember, I told him: just imagine a cabbage with a pen stuck into it. And, for good measure, I added some emotion-related attention to the task. In fact, I said (I was on a roll by now) let's imagine that you really didn't like that over-cooked cabbage that they served for the hospital lunches, so you repeatedly stab the cabbage with a pen, saying 'Die, cabbage, die!' (I added some 'Psycho'-style stabbing gestures for extra effect). He liked that approach. Bingo, on every recall trial after that, Peter remembered the cabbage-pen pair perfectly, and was clearly not classically amnesic. So: circumstantial evidence of executive impairment on several tests, and a demonstration that an external intervention of executive function could remediate dysexecutive memory impairment. I was feeling rather pleased with myself.

All I needed to do was write the case up. But before I did that, it seemed appropriate to take it back for supervision. The next day, I laid the case out: a patient with a long-standing psychiatric disorder; recent deterioration in function, caused by a possible neurological disorder; no signs of impairment in basic cognitive functions; but clear evidence of difficulties with higher level executive function. Probably a pathological process involving the frontal lobes? What were the options? As I'd been trained to do, I worked through the major categories of disease: No sudden onset, so stroke or trauma seemed unlikely. The wrong age group for a likely degenerative disease (as they are usually early or late onset). Some sort of toxic, metabolic or infectious disease seemed possible? Or neoplasm – some sort of frontal tumour? We would probably need that scan?

The next 20 minutes of the supervision – and of my life – were very difficult, and progressively more unpleasant, as my worldview gradually shifted. The downhill path started with my supervisor asking lots of questions about the medical information. Information that I *already* knew about, but which I had conveniently forgotten, or glossed over, in my haste to make the case for executive impairment. If it *was* a stroke, or a tumour, or something toxic, metabolic or infectious, then why were the pupils normal, and the optic fundi, and the reflexes? Why no hard-neurological signs? In fact, the more we talked through the major categories of medical disease, the less likely *any* of them appeared.

There was an especially difficult minute or two in the middle of this conversation, in which I wanted to protest that we couldn't be excluding *every* one of these disease types, because – *couldn't my supervisor see* – the patient was clearly dysexecutive! And so, it gradually dawned on me: the most likely explanation was that the patient probably had *none* of the major categories of medical disease . . . except a psychiatric disorder.

There followed a long slow trudge to the library (in the days before Google Scholar), followed by several hours of immersion in a literature which I had previously not known about: impairment in executive function in psychiatric patients. This was found for *lots* of different kinds of psychiatric disorder, and on many of different measures of executive function (for reviews, see Dibben et al., 2009; Polak et al., 2012; Schillerstrom et al., 2003). None of the impairments were profound, but in general terms, patients with psychiatric disorders – as diverse as psychosis and depression – tended do poorly on executive tasks. Perhaps because it was in the nature of those with psychosis or clinical depression to be distractable, or to have difficultly engaging fully in tackling complex problems? That didn't mean that psychiatric patients *couldn't* have neurological disorders. But it did mean that I was going to have to provide much better evidence for neuropsychological impairment before double pathology became likely, and the neuropsychological evidence was going to have to dove-tail much better with the other medical findings, especially those of my neurologist colleagues.

The other outcome of my error was a flag about over-confidence. In retrospect, one major cause of my mistake had been my feeling so pleased about my assessment of executive function. I felt that knew my stuff, and in showing off I'd been caught up in the operational aspects of the job that I felt I was good at. But successfully identifying executive impairment is not the same as making a diagnostic comment about neuropathology. Like many early career clinicians, I was so caught up in gathering the evidence, and the challenge of deciding which test to administer next, that I'd forgotten the bigger picture. I would probably have been better served by going to the hospital canteen afterwards, and thinking the case through while sipping a cup of their undrinkable coffee. Then I would have understood that the test scores are *not* the diagnosis – not until they fit into the rest of the medical jigsaw puzzle. However, the experience made it clear that I would never again assess a psychiatric patient in the same way.

4. Reflection

The most important thing I remembered from this experience could be captured in a pithy comment that I had heard from Kevin Walsh. It was something that I'd even jotted down in my notes, but up until then I had just not properly understood. Walsh's celebrated phrase is: 'There is no such thing as a neuropsychological test' (Walsh, 1992, p. 122). This little aphorism is often startling when trainees hear it for the first time, and can be just as surprising when deployed to professional colleagues who have little experience of neuropsychology. After all, neuropsychological assessment is all *about* tests, so how can there not be *any* neuropsychological tests? The distinction, of course, is the difference between neuropsychological *test* and neuropsychological *assessment*. As Walsh's phrase elliptically suggests, there are no *neuro*psychological tests, because the only measures which neuropsychologists deploy are *psychological* tests.

There is a widely held – and in many ways dangerously reasonable – assumption that these tests are measures of the psychological processes that appear on the labels and instruction manuals of the glossy tests. Thus, so-called visuo-spatial tests are plainly *designed* to measure visuo-spatial abilities. In such test design, there is always an implication that the test *specifically* targets visuo-spatial processes: that is, that performance centrally requires visuo-spatial ability. This 'specificity' argument seems superficially reasonable, and is indeed true, in many respects. But there is also an implication that the measure *selectively* targets visuo-spatial processes: that is, that performance requires *only* visuo-spatial ability. This implication may be quite unreasonable: for example, because good test performance also requires a degree of memory, attention, visuo-motor or executive function skill, not to mention the language ability required to understand the instructions.

In the hands of a beginner neuropsychologist (or when a fellow professional reads a neuropsychological report), there is a temptation to assume that failure on the test means that the psychological process that appears on the test's front cover must be the what is impaired. This is often followed by the most dangerous caveat: that the cause of test failure is damage to the brain structures that mediate this process. So the patient failed the test of recent episodic memory; therefore, the lesion is in brain regions that underpin recent episodic memory (most obviously, medial temporal lobes and Papez circuit). Similar arguments, at least in a simple form, would apply to tests of language ability and the left convexity (or peri-Sylvian cortex), or to measures of executive function and the frontal lobes.

However, as Peter's case made frighteningly clear, psychological tests can be failed for any number of reasons, including impairments of attention or sustained concentration, failure to properly understand the instructions, or even through intentional choices not to deploy full effort (including insufficient effort, or what used to be described as malingering).

Viewed in this way, the administration of psychological tests – even to neurological patients – need *not* in itself be *neuro*psychological. The *neuro* element is added by the neuropsychologist in many different ways: in choosing the tests based on a neurologically plausible hypothesis; in modifying tests to assess the neuropsychological hypothesis; in noting the qualitative ways in which the patient fails the test; in observing the patients outside the test setting, and mapping this to the reports of family and friends; and, of course, in linking together these findings in the context of the history and relevant medical findings. In all of these ways, there is so much value added by the neuropsychologist to the *neuro* side of the equation. But this neurological element is not captured by the tests themselves, despite their glamorous labels and booklets implying: 'This test measures process x'.

For this reason, Peter's case made me suddenly realise that Walsh's phrase was not only beautifully concise, but that it had a second half – a conclusion that was implicitly *understood* by professional neuropsychologists, but not generally spoken aloud. As the quote opening this chapter records: 'Only the *method* of drawing inferences about tests is neuropsychological' (Walsh, 1992, p. 122, *italics added*). It was an embarrassing lesson to learn. But lessons associated with powerful emotion are all the better recalled, and the memory of this one hasn't faded in 30 years.

And what of Peter? I returned to the referring psychiatrist, clutching a pile of scientific papers on executive function in psychiatric disorders. I explained why I believed that Peter probably did not have a neurological disorder in addition to his psychiatric difficulties. There was a day or two of consideration from the psychiatrist, who then ordered a scan anyway – probably on the better-safe-than sorry argument. It came back, as we might have predicted, within normal limits. If you squinted the right way, there was some minor ventricular enlargement, of the sort that was often reported in cases of chronic schizophrenia. However, that seems less the case in better controlled studies (see Kuo & Pogue-Geile, 2019 for review).

I didn't have much more to do with the case, though I bumped into Peter about six months later, when he had returned from another appointment with the psychiatrist. He was doing as well (or as badly) as he had been when I assessed him. Certainly, his psychiatrist never returned to let us know that we had missed something of neurological importance, so I assume that we made the correct diagnosis. I never saw Peter again, but I think about him every time that I see a patient with a psychiatric disorder, but who does badly on measures of executive function. And I think about him when I walk down the aisle of a supermarket, and pass the section selling water filters.

References

Bentall, R.P. (2003). *Madness explained: Psychosis and human nature*. London: Penguin.

Dibben, C.R.M., Rice, C., Laws, K. & McKenna, P.J. (2009). Is executive impairment associated with schizophrenic syndromes? A meta-analysis. *Psychological Medicine*, 39, 381–392.

Kuo, S.S. & Pogue-Geile, M.F. (2019). Variation in fourteen brain structure volumes in schizophrenia: A comprehensive meta-analysis of 246 studies. *Neuroscience and Biobehavioural Reviews*, 98, 85–94.

Polak, A.R., Witteveen, A.B., Reitsma, J.B. & Olff, M. (2012). The role of executive function in posttraumatic stress disorder: A systematic review. *Journal of Affective Disorders*, 141, 11–21.

Schillerstrom, J.E., Deuter, M.S., Wyatt, R., Stern, S.L. & Royall, D.R. (2003). Prevalence of executive impairment in patients seen by a psychiatry consultation service. *Psychosomatics*, 44(4), 290–297.

Walsh, K.W. (1992). Some gnomes worth knowing. *Clinical Neuropsychologist*, 6(2), 119–133.

Note

1 Those familiar with the literature on developmental experience and serious mental illness will be familiar with accounts like this of family history and psychiatric disorder. There is a vast literature demonstrating the role played by adverse early childhood experiences, poor parental mental health, being a member of an oppressed or disadvantaged community, high levels of 'expressed emotion' in family setting, and the like. These (and a range of other variables) are risk factors not only for the likelihood of *developing* mental illness, but also play a role in *sustaining* mental illness in those who are already sufferers. For a readable account of this enormous literature, Richard Bentall's (2003) *Madness Explained* might be a useful introduction.

4   Absence of evidence

Rudi Coetzer

'Every normal person, in fact, is only normal on the average'.

—Sigmund Freud

1. Situation

All too often in the mundane routine of daily clinics in neurology and neuro-surgery departments, the clinical neuropsychologist habituates to seeing large numbers of patients with unequivocal brain damage. Patients have clear cognitive impairment, which gradually already reveals itself during the bedside assessment. This preliminary assessment almost serves purely for generating the main hypotheses to be considered during formal neuropsychological testing. Inevitably though, the formal neuropsychological testing reveals even more obvious evidence of the presence of cognitive impairment. In these cases, brain imaging findings are rarely normal. It can be very much a world of black and white. Almost without exception, the neuropsychologist can one way or another somehow 'fit' the cognitive profile identified with neuropsychological testing to the lesion (or lesions) as reported by the neuroradiologists.

There is something of an art to this. The interconnectivity of cognitive functions in the human brain makes it possible for the less experienced clinical neuropsychologist to reason that an almost infinite number of profiles of neuropsychological impairment could just possibly, or sometimes even almost definitely, be compatible with an equally large number of scan abnormalities. This is perhaps because it is unusual to see anybody *without* some form of brain injury or illness in these settings. Also, the patients that neuropsychologists see are typically those who have already been *diagnosed* with neurological abnormalities. It follows that they will almost certainly have cognitive impairment. We simply don't receive referrals for people with whom nothing (neurologically) is wrong.

2. Example

The day, or at least the morning, once I was actually inside the hospital, was uneventful. At the ward round there were, rather unusually, only two referrals for neuropsychology. And both were for neuropsychological testing. The first

DOI:10.4324/9781003300748-4

patient had sustained a severe traumatic brain injury just over a month previously, but was now considered well enough to go home later in the week. The neurosurgery ward needed a baseline cognitive assessment before he could go. Straightforward, I thought. Which it did turn out to be. I saw the patient with the TBI first, to facilitate the discharge process in case he was to go home that day. So the next patient, for the afternoon, was Dan.

Dan came from a suburb near the hospital, and was seen in outpatients. He was neatly dressed, friendly and seemed pretty relaxed when I went to collect him in the waiting room. He had short hair, a firm handshake (with his right hand, I noted) and lively green eyes. Quite tall, lean, looks like he may be a sportsman, or possibly work with his hands. He was 43 years old, and has been referred for testing, according to a scribble in the clinic diary. No surprises there then. Dan follows me to my office further down the corridor. I can hear his trainers making rhythmic, even, squeaky sounds on the shiny green vinyl floor, the auditory mirror of a normal gait.

We start at the beginning. I ask if he is experiencing any problems at present. Dan replies that he is fine, but a bit busy at work. Which he says he is grateful for. Dan is a technician, and self-employed. He tells me that he lost quite a bit of income due to his recent hospital stay. I ask what he was in hospital for. Dan says he had a stroke. I cannot help but wonder what type of stroke this might have been? From our relatively brief interaction, I cannot, for the life of me, detect any obvious physical or perceptual impairment. Actually, never mind obvious, there is not even a subtle sign. No facial asymmetry, or slight weakness, no change in gait, visual or hearing difficulties, or anything else I can see? How strange.

What were his symptoms when he had the stroke, I enquire. Dan tells me that he was straining to move a heavy fridge to gain access to the back. Next thing everything went black. He cannot remember from there on. From what he was told, the owner of the house found him on the kitchen floor and called an ambulance. Dan was taken to hospital, but remembers nothing of the journey. He tells me that he understands that he was seen by the doctors, who 'fixed' his stroke. His first memory is of waking up 'in a strange white room'. Dan soon figured out that he was in hospital, and thought he must have had a heart attack. He felt a bit fatigued for a few days while in hospital, but quickly got his strength back. He was told by the doctors that everything was fine, that there would be no further strokes. He went for follow-up a month later, and was again told that, from their point of view, the problem was 'fixed'. But just to be on the safe side, he would be referred for tests in about six months. I am not quite sure if this refers to his appointment with me?

I don't quite understand what exactly Dan's problem, if anything, is. He tells me not only that he had a stroke, and there is a referral, but also that he does not really have any problems? It will probably all come out in the wash? The history, that is. As clinicians, we live or die by taking a history, and by now I believe I can do as thorough a history as any other clinical neuropsychologist.

I start taking down the developmental milestones. Dan was born locally, with no complications, and his early development was entirely normal. He had lots of friends and socialised well at school. I catch myself thinking that this probably reflects very truthfully his personality as an adult also. Dan is very pleasant, engages well with the assessment situation, and not infrequently cracks a joke as well – socially skilled, outgoing and likable.

As I continue with finding out a bit more about Dan, my thoughts become a bit clearer. This man does not present like someone who has had *any* major brain injury or illness, I decide. It was time to form some preliminary hypotheses, and potentially save myself a lot of work. I wonder if he might have fainted, or blacked out? I quickly discard this as ridiculous. Surely nobody in a major academic teaching hospital would ever refer a patient with a history of fainting for neuropsychological testing. Much more likely something like a Transient Ischaemic Attack. They typically resolve in well under 24 hours, so would perfectly explain everything? And explain why the neuropsychological testing seemed so normal?

I want to take no chances, so we continue with the history: because evidence, especially evidence integrated from different sources such as the history, is everything in case formulation. Dan achieved two A-levels, and continued to complete a diploma in engineering. After qualifying from a technical college in the city, he started a short apprenticeship to specialise, before deciding to work for himself, rather than with a big company. He now fixes household appliances. There's more money and freedom in this, he says, and he further qualifies this by saying he doesn't like working for a boss. He is married and has two kids. There is no history of mental health difficulties, and he tells me he has never been admitted to a psychiatric hospital. Dan is quite specific on this, and I note that he spontaneously names the three main local psychiatric hospitals. How is he so familiar with their exact, formal names I ask? Oh, he has fixed some of their stoves and fridges in their kitchens, he tells me. We cover his family history, which reveals nothing of interest. Diplomatically I enquire about substance misuse. Nothing. Not even a little bit of alcohol, I gently probe. Dan smiles and says he occasionally has a drink over weekends, but that it's not really his thing. He acknowledges that this is probably hard to believe though, and laughs. I reassure Dan that I believe him.

Before we conclude the history, I ask Dan about head injuries. I make it clear that I mean only any injuries resulting in loss of consciousness, and requiring admission to hospital – in other words, traumatic brain injury, not 'Friday night fights'. Never had anything like that, he tells me. I have increasingly come to realise there is absolutely nothing in his history, and a bit of doubt sets in. The absence of any evidence of a brain injury or illness is unusual in this job. To double check, I ask about concussion. The most to be found here is the odd banging of his head against an appliance door while working. Dan winks, and tells me that he never even saw stars. His scalp is clearly visible because of his short hair, and he has no scars on his head, and definitely not any signs of recent (or even remote) neurosurgery.

Having exhausted all the neurological factors I thought could be relevant to his case, I change my angle, and ask if he has any stress at work, or any other things that worry him. Dan laughs, and says that there is actually nothing bothering him, and that one could say his life is possibly just a bit boring. The history is certainly clear, I decide, but I have a feeling that I should be extra careful and observant when doing the clinical assessment. I start with the bedside cognitive testing, even though Dan has been booked for formal neuropsychological testing. Relying too heavily on tests can be a very high-risk strategy, I have by now learnt. We can all too easily be seduced by numbers and percentiles, and lulled into the false sense that because we have numerical data, which we might regard (incorrectly) as better evidence.

Today, the bedside testing yields nothing useful for forming new hypotheses to be considered during the neuropsychology testing proper. Dan is fully orientated for time, place and person. His performance on brief tests of concentration and attention is fine. There are no obvious, or even minor, speech or language problems. He easily retains and recalls three words after 15 minutes. Copying the Necker cube poses no problems to Dan. Tells me he is good at technical drawings, because of the nature of his work. He sails through mental calculation. Again, he points out that he does this sort of stuff every day in his job. Otherwise, he won't be able to provide customers with on-the-spot quotes for work. I do a few simple executive function tests. He finds these a bit bemusing, from the look of things. But there is no evidence of perseveration, concreteness, poor problem-solving, impulsivity or inability to shift set.

After completing my bedside cognitive assessment, I do a brief mental status examination. Dan makes good eye contact, and his expression of affect to me looks appropriate, and congruent. He is definitely not depressed, nor anxious. Dan tells me that he sleeps well, that his appetite is good, and that he regularly exercises by walking the dog in the evenings. His energy and drive appear fine too. He has not experienced any change in his weight over the past month. Dan's thought processes and perceptual functions are normal. I conclude the clinical assessment and tell Dan that we'll have a break now.

During the short break after the clinical assessment, I send Dan to the hospital canteen to have something to eat and drink. I tell him that when he comes back we will start with the formal neuropsychological testing. When Dan returns, I explain what the testing will entail, and roughly how long it should take. In view of his very good educational and employment achievements, I decide to do a shortened (four subtest) Wechsler Adult Intelligence Scale. I score as we go along. My reasoning so far appears to be correct. Dan scores a pro-rated IQ of 109. And no differences between the two verbal and two nonverbal tests, in fact all four subtests produce very similar standard scores. Memory is the next neuropsychological function I test, using the Wechsler Memory Scale. Dan's performance is above average on Associative Learning, Logical Memory and Visual Reproduction, and almost certainly in keeping with his general cognitive ability. Delayed recall (30 minutes) of the Rey Complex Figure yields another average score. I remind myself that as interns we were told this is a rather difficult visual recall task. And to be aware that it was not unusual for normal controls to occasionally produce sub-optimal scores on this part of the test. Dan's Benton Visual Retention Test performance produces scores well within the norm for his age and general intellectual ability. Dan does not have any sort of memory problem, I decide.

The neuropsychological testing is concluded with briefly looking at Dan's executive control (frontal) functions. His Rey Complex Figure score is above the 90th percentile, but more relevant to the question of executive control function, his strategy is entirely normal. No fragmentation, poor planning or perseveration is to be seen in his copying of the figure. We finish off with some tests to look at executive function, including the Austin Maze and Stroop test. Once again all his test results are normal – and normal when considered against his likely pre-morbid intellectual ability. I decide to send Dan on his way. I will review him in clinic over the next few weeks, but try to reassure him that I did not see any specific, significant or obvious impairments on his neuropsychological test performance today.

When Dan is gone, slight doubt starts to gnaw at the edges of my confidence again. I look over the test results again, and also check my scoring. No errors of calculation. There really is no evidence of impairment on *any* of the tests, and also no qualitative pointers towards neurological injury or illness. I wonder who referred him? Probably a new registrar or house doctor in one of the wards. I go to check with the secretary in our unit's reception. I find out he was referred by neurosurgery, by one of the consultants. That's a bit surprising. I look at our file, and the referral form. It simply asks for testing, and is signed by one of the consultant's juniors. Time to go home early for a change.

But I don't. Even though it's a lovely day outside, and if I were to rush, there would still be time for a walk, in good light, before supper, I don't leave. The doubt has started to bite. An experienced clinical neuropsychologist I knew always told us that 'if things don't add up, they don't add up'. 'A man with a normal brain scan should not have a grossly impaired neuropsychological test profile', another of her favourite sayings. So while packing up on this afternoon, I start to ruminate over why a neurosurgeon would ask for neuropsychological testing of a patient without any cognitive impairment. For a few minutes I worry that I missed something. But then my anxiety and doubt gradually start to subside, and I decide, actually, there is no evidence of cognitive impairment. That means that there really is very little, if any of a major neurological problem. Plus, I did not skimp on the history taking – and clinically, nothing of note either.

Only one way to find out – go up to the ward, and have a look at their file (which has not yet come down to us). 'If things don't add up, they don't add up'. As I enter the ward, and go into the nurses' station, I immediately notice Dr Smith, the neurosurgeon standing by the file trolley. He looks up, smiles and asks how I've been. I reply that everything is good, and crack a joke that he should send more patients without any cognitive impairment to me for testing. It is nice to be on 'light duties' for a change. Dr Smith asks who that might be, and I begin to tell him about Dan's general clinical presentation. He nods knowingly, and asks me what the neuropsychological test results were, and what I made of Dan's presentation.

Dr Smith is a very good listener. I cannot help but notice that he looks like a man who never has to make life and death decisions under unimaginably stressful situations, which must surely regularly occur on the operating table of a brain surgeon. He listens attentively to my whole presentation, and seems genuinely interested. It's not often that one has a captive audience in a neuro-surgeon and I catch myself feeling proud for having this opportunity! At the end of my presentation I summarise the case, pointing out that Dan's history is entirely normal, there was nothing on clinical bedside exam (he's certainly not depressed, I add), and all his psychological tests were in the normal range.

I continue my feedback to Dr Smith. There is no evidence whatsoever of any neuropsychological impairment, and I wondered if Dan suffered fainting spells, or more likely, had a Transient Ischaemic Attack? But if I were to nail my colours to the mast, I add, I think the absence of any neuropsychologi-cal evidence points towards a functional, non-biological aetiology. Dr Smith looked as if he was pondering something, weighing up my first two suggestions of possible explanations of Dan's recent admission to hospital. He also looked really pleased to hear the test results were fine. But he does not seem to have heard, or taken in anything regarding my third hypothesis. I feel reassured, and pleased that neuropsychological assessment could make such a useful contribu-tion to diagnostic formulation in neurosurgery. The day is turning out to be much, much better than it started.

Dr Smith's calm voice pulls me back to the reality of being in the ward. He tells me Dan is a very lucky man to be alive. I am immediately just that little bit less confident, a slight flutter in my chest. Dr Smith tells me Dan had a haem-orrhage in the Circle of Willis – more specifically, the anterior communicating artery of the Circle of Willis. His face now very serious, Dr Smith recounts how Dan came very close to dying on the operating table, but that they man-aged to clip what must surely have been an aneurysm waiting to explode, and then of course did exactly that, necessitating him to be rushed to hospital. Perhaps straining with the heavy fridge was the straw which broke the camel's back, so to speak. Dr Smith continues: Obviously from his perspective as a neurosurgeon, it is extremely good news that I found no cognitive impairment.

Dr Smith continues and points out when it is the anterior communicating artery within the Circle of Willis which causes the mischief – we can see more frontal problems. Which he acknowledges is more difficult to test for, given the structured nature of the testing situation and tests used. Sometimes, one has to look for possible subtle behavioural or personality changes; Dr Smith continues: for example, a very serious person becoming a bit more jocular, or impulsive, or apathetic, and so forth. I can now feel a throbbing sensation in my temples. Was Dan a bit too light hearted, or jocular for a man who had recently suffered a life-threatening illness, I wonder by myself. Dr Smith then smiles, and concludes by saying that I should remember that in healthcare one normal investigation doesn't mean everything else will be normal also. Never mind a CT scan. He should know, he physically saw, and clipped Dan's aneurysm.

3. Error

Dan's case reminds us of some of the seminal work of Teuber. Hans–Lucas Teuber is credited with stating that 'absence of evidence is not evidence of absence' within the neuropsychological context. In Dan's case, this was the big error of clinical reasoning I made. The concept of negative findings not necessarily excluding positive findings has, of course, not only been considered in clinical neuropsychology. For example, Altman and Bland (1995) also caution against falling into the trap of not realising that absence of evidence does not equal evidence of absence (of findings) in a medical statistical context. And, of course, that was exactly what the character of Dr Smith diplomatically pointed out in the case example of Dan. Lezak et al. (2012) discuss the application of Teuber's insight to modern clinical neuropsychological testing, and points out that while an absence of impaired scores is common in cognitively intact persons, this may also occur in clinical populations with known brain damage. The flaw in the clinical neuropsychologist's reasoning about Dan to some extent was the opposite of what most newly qualified clinical neuropsychologists tend to make – assuming abnormal test scores simply must mean the presence of an abnormal brain scan. Perhaps the opposite situation that of finding a normal test protocol in someone who looked 'totally normal' as well resulted in a 'blindside' mistake in my clinical reasoning.

4. Reflection

Neuropsychological testing can produce a profile of scores that are all within a normal range, and for a few different reasons (see also Lezak et al., 2012). Sometimes the testing might have been too limited in range. In other situations, the specific tests, which *might* have detected a deficit, were not administered. Furthermore, tests vary in their sensitivity to detect impairment. Most importantly, there is also the issue of persons with high levels of general cognitive ability, or pre-morbid intelligence. They have substantial cognitive reserve, and after an acquired brain injury are able to mask specific neuropsychological impairments. With the best will in the world, the clinical neuropsychologist is unlikely to get the predicted premorbid IQ quite right. Yet this is crucial, as premorbid IQ provides the context of 'norming to the individual', which lies at the heart of interpretation.

Other than technical issues related to neuropsychological testing, there is also the additional problem of confirmation bias. Once I started to hypothesise that Dan's presentation, history and test results all pointed to the *absence* of any major neurological illness or injury, I increasingly became less and less open to alternative explanations for his presentation. In effect, I found more and more evidence for *my* hypothesis. Although test results and other data in neuropsychology are objective, the interaction of the clinician with their patients is still akin to being the subjective canvas, where these test data will be painted into the whole of a picture. No wonder clinical neuropsychology is both science and art!

The best advice then is: Read the referral. If you find nothing, go off and try to discover more information about the patient's medical history, and especially around the incident that caused their recent brain injury. There is all too often material there that is *not* covered in the referral letter.

Later that night I went to read a bit more about haemorrhages and aneurysms linked to the Circle of Willis. Neurosurgical access was traditionally through the bones of the lateral surface of the skull (i.e. the frontal, temporal and parietal), in the same way that surgeons find access to drain a subdural. Surgery was also performed via the nasal cavity, leaving no visible scarring on the cranium. This procedure has, of course, now changed, with adoption of endovascular coiling, with entry from the femoral artery, leaving even fewer traces.

What then of the neuropsychological findings that I might have expected? Cognitive impairment after Circle of Willis aneurysms can include memory problems (new learning and retention) given its proximity to various subcortical structures, particularly the limbic system. But executive problems are not uncommon, and are thought to be the result of the disruption of basal striatal cortical pathways to the prefrontal cortex. For this reason, personality changes are reported too after Circle of Willis aneurysms and bleeds. As ever, these are best observed by performing collateral interviews, with relatives or other persons who knew the patient well prior to their brain injury.

It all made me think of Lezak et al. (2012) reminder that 'normal' performance might be a result of testing that was too limited in range. That there are tests which *might* have detected a deficit but were not administered.

I never saw Dan again. But the idea of 'might have detected' often makes me think about Dan's jokes. So, the next time I face a Circle of Willis haemorrhage, I would administer several additional tests of executive control function. Importantly, I would better use my qualitative observations of behaviours during the consultation. And speak to a relative? Definitely. As the quote that opens this chapter suggests, I would always try to remember that in the final analysis 'normality' is relative.

References

Altman, D. G. & Bland, J. M. (1995). Absence of evidence is not evidence of absence. *British Medical Journal*, (311): 485.

Lezak, M. D., Howieson, D. B., Bigler, E. D. & Tranel, D. (2012). *Neuropsychological Assessment* (5th edition). Oxford University Press.

5 Problematic pyramids

Oliver Turnbull

'For in disease the most voluntary or most special movements, faculties etc., suffer first and most, that is in an order the exact opposite of evolution'.
—John Hughlings Jackson

1. Situation

The cornerstone of neuropsychological assessment is differential performance – or perhaps more accurately, *patterns* of differential performance. Pre- versus post-morbid, immediate versus recent memory, receptive versus expressive language . . . and of course patient versus neurologically normal controls. We evaluate a deficit, and we try to judge whether it is a 'real' deficit: Is it that different from pre-morbid performance? Is this kind of impaired (recent) memory better than the expected kind of intact (immediate) memory? How many standard deviations from the group mean is the patient's score? This is the standard fare of any module on neuropsychological assessment, with all the talk of Scaled Scores, and correction for age or years of education. You can't become a clinical neuropsychologist without knowing this meaning of differential performance. And it's reasonably easy to achieve, because (at least in theory, as discussed in other chapters) the label on the outside of the box tells you what the test assesses: this test for recent memory, and that for immediate memory.

But there is another form of 'differential', which the label on the box doesn't tell you about: when *one* psychological ability or skill can be assessed using two *different* psychological processes. How can that happen? It happens because of a pyramid: complex psychological processes are built on simpler ones, typically *several* simpler ones, so that there is more than one way to assess the more complex skill. And the most complex psychological process is, of course, executive function. No domain of mental life taxes the assessment skills of the clinician more, and that increases the need to be vigilant about making errors. But this sort of error isn't one that tends to be described in the average neuropsychological assessment module, and it's not going to be solved by understanding Gaussian distributions, or test-retest reliability. Instead, it can only be understood by realising that any test of executive function has to be built on basic cognitive components. Broad categories might be object recognition, language

DOI:10.4324/9781003300748-5

or memory. And, importantly, to understand that, all too often, executive measures are built on several more foundational skills.

This could all be solved if there was a simple chart that showed the beginner clinician what this mapping of executive measure to foundational skill looks like. However, there is (in our experience) no such chart. Indeed, there would be technical barriers to generating one. As a result, trainees often aren't aware of this as a confounding issue – that is, until they make a diagnostic error, and are reminded about the mistake by their supervisor. Then, strangely enough, they realise that they knew the fundamentals of this problem all along. But they hadn't consciously been aware of it as a trap-door. This is a case that illustrates the heart of the problem.

2. Example

The one thing that I was sure about was that Sion had suffered a severe closed head injury. I'd followed his progress most of the way through the system, which started with seeing him when he was on a ventilator in Neurosurgery, in the days following his motorcycle accident. There was no assessing him then, of course. But I knew that the longer he was lying in our Intensive Care Unit, the more likely I was – unfortunately – to be finding something of neuropsychological interest when he regained consciousness. Over the course of a few weeks, he gradually emerged up the ladder of the Glasgow Coma Scale: at first silent and intubated, then incomprehensible and noisy; gradually more comprehensible, but still noisy; then a little less noisy, but still rather rude – at least by the standards of polite dinner party conversation. I checked in with him for a few minutes when I was in Neurosurgery, and it was clear that the Post Traumatic Amnesia (PTA) was looking like a few weeks in duration. Of course, this didn't bode well – this one would be in the 'fingers crossed' domain.

A few weeks later, and after a lot of haggling between services, Sion appeared in our rehabilitation hospital – where I was the same trainee, wearing a slightly different hat. By now, the worst of the disinhibition seemed to have recovered – but there was still far too much bad language for him to be invited to any dinner parties. And not just bad language: if this had been a work rather than a hospital environment, then Sion would probably have been eligible for a sexual harassment case. The nursing staff handled it with good grace, as ever. But anyone could see that Sion was a very long way from going back to his job as a University Lecturer in biology.

I was delaying a more formal neuropsychological assessment for a while yet, to allow for more recovery. There was no point in trying to formally assess someone whose attention span was only a few seconds. But I tried to keep regular tabs on his basic memory function, looking for a period when he would be able to form decent episodic memories for consecutive days. Then I could declare PTA over. There was one difficult moment in which I'd talked to his wife about 'Sion's PTA', which of course I meant as Post Traumatic Amnesia. But then his wife had asked about what his recovery had to do with the Parent Teacher Association? I made a mental note to try and avoid acronyms when speaking to family. Alas, it wasn't the worst mistake I'd make with Sion's assessment.

Actually, it was increasingly looking as if I wasn't speaking to Sion's wife, so much as his soon-to-be *ex*-wife. It turned out that a degree of marital breakdown had been on the cards for quite a while, perhaps linked to the same midlife crisis that had seen Sion buy the motorcycle. And so my discussions with her about Sion's recovery had also made me realise that she had a huge dilemma: leave a marriage that was plainly in an even worse state than before the accident . . . or stay with her husband, because society tends to frown on those who leave their spouses when they have just been hospitalised. This was my first encounter with the dilemma, which I later discovered was all too common for the partners of neurological patients. So, I remembered my psychotherapy lectures, listened to her and tried not to take sides: Sion's wife had enough on her plate without marital advice from a 20-something trainee.

However, saving Sion's marriage, or addressing his wife's grief and distress, was not my central concern. Time, in any rehabilitation unit, is a precious commodity, and a key part of my job was to assess Sion as a neuropsychologist, and offer some advice to the multi-disciplinary team about how this might shape the various aspects of his rehabilitation. I had done this several times for patients with closed head injury, and the answer had always been a variant on the theme of executive dysfunction. The pathological basis of this had been clear to me from the start of my training: ever since the memorable moment in my brain dissection class when our lecturer was describing the anatomy of the base of the skull. The division between the anterior and middle cranial fossae features a huge plummeting step, down the wing of the sphenoid bone. It forms a ridge that could remind you of the edge of Niagara Falls . . . but sharper. The lecturer encouraged us to pass the skull around, and to run our fingers across that sharp little ridge – something I still ask our students to do when I teach neuroanatomy classes today.

I follow this up with a small lesson on how the anterior and middle cranial fossae hold the frontal and temporal lobes, both of which become so badly contused when the brain decelerates inside the cranial cavity: as both lobes are stretched and torn by the bony edges. Whenever I teach this material, I tell my students to think about the pathology – and especially whenever they might be tempted to take risks when driving their own cars. And I always wonder whether that small thought might have saved one or two lives over the years? Alas, the lesson was too late for Sion. He might have been a Lecturer in biology, but the University biology curriculum probably didn't cover the anatomy of the base of the skull, nor its relationship to closed head injury. Regardless, this bit of anatomy explained why so many of our closed head injury patients had orbital frontal contusions, and showed why their chronic outcome was so dysexecutive. My main job was going to be establishing which *sorts* of dysexecutive.

3. Error

Across a few sessions, I administered a range of basic executive function measures. I was careful not to do them all at once, given that Sion was distractable, and prone to tiredness, so it seemed best to work in batches. One element of his executive abilities was coming out especially clearly, and probably didn't need any formal measures: Sion was clearly disinhibited. My report was going to document this with a few qualitative descriptions of socially inappropriate comments, of rule breaking during tests, and by failure to stay on task as a result of distraction. And I topped this up with some scores on a 'Go, no-go' task, and a fairly poor performance on the Stroop test. So bad, in fact, that I sometimes wondered whether he was even reading down the word list sequentially?

That was the easy bit, but not especially laudable. None of the nurses or rehabilitation therapists was going to give me much credit for discovering that a man who commented daily on women's breast-size showed features of disinhibition. I needed to add some value. And so his problem-solving ability, one of the other key domains of executive function, seemed a good place to investigate. So, I picked a few other measures. Perhaps the Rey-Osterrieth Complex Figure? He drew that catastrophically, in a really a disorganised way. Block Design? Again, really terrible. And the Austin Maze? He couldn't even begin to learn the route, though a quick addition of Story Recall showed that he wasn't amnesic. So I was on to something with the problem-solving issues.

The one minor concern was that the problem-solving argument didn't seem to apply to *all* of the measures of executive function. On the Cognitive Estimates task, he seemed much better – within normal limits, actually, with some nice examples of hypothesis-testing and drawing conclusions. But he had probably been a clever chap pre-morbidly? And his ability to explain Proverbs was also rather impressive, with some of abstract thinking. Still, that was enough for me – poor performance on three of my five executive tasks was a decent result. I remembered from my lectures on the frontal lobes that executive function performance could be variable, and that the tests were poorly inter-correlated, so finding evidence on a *majority* of the tasks seemed evidence enough. So, I had a clear conclusion. . . . Sion had difficulties in two quite distinct domains of executive function: he was disinhibited and he had impaired problem-solving.

I'd also remembered another clinical fundamental: linking together my hypothesis of neuropsychological impairment with the rest of the medical findings. Formulation is the fancy term for it. Did my 'two kinds of executive impairment' argument match what we knew about neuropathology? Absolutely. The one thing we could be sure about was that Sion had a serious head injury. The substantial duration of PTA predicted that. And the fundamentals of sphenoid ridges, and deceleration-related-contusion, made him perfectly entitled to frontal lesions and executive impairment. Could this be confirmed more precisely on scan? That was less clear. I knew that one needed to review scan results with caution in closed head injury – doubly so back then, when the technology was so fuzzy. Much of the tearing of axons, and the shearing injuries on the grey-white matter boundary, were microscopic – and often impossible to detect on scan. But I had a good long look at Sion's frontal lobes from the radiologist's scan. Perhaps I was imagining some of it – but there clearly seemed to be several areas of frontal gliosis, bilaterally. Another important clinical conclusion ticked off the list, even if a little imprecisely.

At this stage, there was at least one potential warning light that I might have noticed – one which has recurred throughout many of these narratives. It's one thing to establish poor test performance on a measure of psychological function, but the alert clinician should always be seeking to tie the test performance to *other* sources of evidence, to triangulate information. It is particularly important here to gather information from those who spend more time with the patient, and see patients functioning in more ecologically valid environments: family members, friends or indeed therapists. The staff were quite clear about Sion's disinhibition, of course. He had quite a reputation for that on the ward. But there was no feedback from them about the problem-solving issue. Not too surprising, perhaps, given that hospital wards are structured places. Mealtimes and visiting hours are scheduled for the patient, and a therapist would come to the ward to meet their patient for a session, or a porter would deliver them to the therapy room. So there weren't too many new or uncertain situations that demanded complex problem-solving skills, apart from my executive tests.

Another useful source of corroborating evidence would be the behaviour of the patient in the test setting, but outside of formal test performance. What was the Sion's behaviour like during the history taking? How easily had he understood the various test instructions? What did he do between tests, or how easily did his attention wander off during a test? How did he relate to the examiner? Here, again, there was lots of evidence of disinhibition: Sion had made a few fairly childish jokes, and his attention had often wandered. But yet again, evidence of a problem-solving impairment, or of concrete thinking, was absent. Sion had spoken for a while across his various assessment sessions, and covered a range number of topics, thanks to his disinhibition and wandering attention. But, in retrospect, the content of those discussions was often far from concrete. He had opinions on politics and the corruption of government officials, on the decline of morals in the young (a little ironic, given the common target of his disinhibition), and on the causes of poor performance of his football team, by virtue of poor strategic choices of their manager. He also had expressed an opinion on his possible return to work – one that was surprisingly accurate. He said with reasonable insight that he *felt* confident that he could manage, but he could see that others would find his behaviour inappropriate. So, on balance, perhaps the right time hadn't arrived yet, he felt. Quite insightful, actually?

In short, he often had the abstract and strategic perspective on the world that one might expect from someone with *intact* executive function, except that his wandering attention meant that he wouldn't follow a conversational strand for long. But when he was in that zone, he was a clever man, and as erudite and intellectual as one could reasonably hope for. I realised this in retrospect, of course. At the time, I was dazzled by the poor set of test performances, and firmly on the path of impairments in both inhibition and problem-solving.

And so I was off for my weekly supervision – armed with a range of test scores, and a clear hypothesis. The bulk of the supervision went very well. Yes, Sion had a serious head injury. Yes, I seemed correct about PTA. Yes, I had been correct in waiting for the confusional state to lift before formally assessing him. Yes, the scan might well suggest frontal contusions, and he was entitled to executive impairment. Yes, the linking of things around his disinhibition seemed clear: in reports from staff, in the behaviour in the test setting with me, and indeed on the formal measures of inhibition themselves. It was looking good.

Alas, the conversation took a troubling turn when it came to the question of the problem-solving impairment. It started with the list of failed tests, and the ratio of failed to pass. Serious failure on the Rey Figure, Block Design and the Austin Maze seemed clear – on the other hand, they pass on Cognitive Estimates and Proverbs. In retrospect, I think I presented some sort of 'averaging' argument: as one might do when working out someone's final degree classification, or earnings across a few months of patchy part-time work. Sion fails three out of five tests very badly. Sion does fairly well on the other two. So, on balance, this is a fail.

With the benefit of hindsight, this argument seems hard to defend, and for several reasons. One key element is the assumption that all five of the tests are measuring the same thing. Based on the argument described earlier, it might seem that all *are*: each of the five is (amongst other things) a measure of executive function, and all are (to varying degrees) loaded on the problem-solving element. That is, of course, what it says on the box? But, as the experienced neuropsychologist will know, the problem is that all psychological measures have loadings on *several* psychological functions – an argument that applies especially to tests of executive function. More importantly, any pattern of differential performance between tests should be thought through, and hypothesis-tested, rather than simply brushed under the carpet. And, heaven knows, Sion had quite a pattern of differential performance.

And so my supervisor started asking questions about the tests: questions that I mostly knew the answers to, though perhaps I didn't want to hear them. Did the poor problem-solving and abstract thinking test performance match the reports of family and staff, and did it match his behaviour in the assessment setting? Er . . . no, it didn't really. Was there evidence for widespread frontal contusions on scan, especially involving the dorso-lateral surface, not simply the ventral surface? Er . . . not exactly. And finally, the question that floored me: was there anything about the Rey Figure, Block Design and the Austin Maze, which made them categorically different to Cognitive Estimates and Proverbs? I couldn't think. Or at least I couldn't think clearly, with the spotlight so clearly on me.

So, could I please describe, in words of one syllable, what the Rey Figure, Block Design and the Austin Maze consisted of, as measures? Sure: in one you copy a complicated figure, in another you arrange some blocks to match a complicated pattern, and in the next, you learn a complicated route round a maze. And what did they all have in common, apart from the fact that (like all measures of executive function) they were complicated? Er . . . surely that not all of them needed recent memory? And then the penny dropped . . . all of them were measures of visuo-spatial ability!

And, in words of one syllable, what were Cognitive Estimates and Proverbs? One was judgements about complicated questions that no-one knew the pre-cise answers to. And the other was an abstract understanding of proverbs? And they had in common . . . ? The landscape was starting to become worryingly clear. They were both primarily *verbal* measures.

And so, in one small minute, the landscape had changed. Why had Sion failed only the *executive* tests that loaded on *visuo-spatial* ability? A long pause, and a deep breath . . . the most plausible hypothesis, unfortunately for me, was that he had a visuo-spatial impairment. So . . . had I administered any other measures of visuo-spatial ability, said my supervisor? Well no . . . because I had assumed that, like my previous patients with closed head injury, Steven would simply be dysexecutive. And, my supervisor added, if he *did* have a visuo-spatial deficit, where might one look for the patient to have a brain lesion? Some-where posterior, probably parietal, or parieto-temporal, or the like . . . prob-ably right-lateralised? And did Steven have any parieto-temporal lesions on scan? Er . . . I wasn't sure. Why? Because? Because I hadn't looked at the scan? And then a pause. Actually . . . I *had* looked at the scan. But because when I read the scan, I'd only really been looking at his frontal lobes.

4. Reflection

Why had I painted myself into this corner? For several reasons. The most important had been not understanding the 'pyramid' structure of psychologi-cal skills, and their particular relevance to measures of executive function. It's an undergraduate truism to say that cognitive processes are complex – and every undergraduate course in cognitive psychology is littered with the box and arrow flow-chart diagrams to prove it. The higher-level executive skills sit at the top of this pyramid: establishing the nature of the problem, identifying goals, setting the necessary sub-goals and working out which basic cognitive skills are required to achieve them.

But what will happen if one of those *basic* cognitive skills is impaired? The goal isn't achieved, and the pyramid falls. But the reason for the failure might not be because the executive ability is *itself* impaired, but because the founda-tional skill is absent. As has been discussed elsewhere, even if the label on the test *says* executive function, there are ways for the patient with *normal* execu-tive function to fail. In the case of Sion, it was possible that poor visuo-spatial skill was producing failure on spatially loaded executive measures, but allowing normal performance on the more linguistically based tests. The data allowing me to draw this inference were all there for me to *see*, but I hadn't been *looking*.

This error forces us to seriously consider two relatively old and critical concepts in clinical neuropsychology. The first is a *qualitative* analysis of the disorder, and the second a process approach. These concepts are perhaps the best tools we have to deal with the recurrent issues brought about by problematic pyramids. Both concepts do not relate to whether the patient *fails* a test. There are many ways to fail a test – but more importantly—*how* they fail the test, or how they fail to master the task. If we look at (say) the Rey-Osterrieth Figure, there are several ways in which a patient can obtain an impaired score. Components might be put together in a tidy spatial fashion, with all the main features of the figure, but the patient forgets, or misplaces, important internal details. Here, the core failure is some sort of sloppiness in performance (of various cause), or poor planning. Other patients, like our Sion, can struggle orienting individual lines, and co-locating pieces of the figure in order to build a whole, suggesting a difficulty in manipulating objects within space.

In both cases, the same *tasks* are failed, but for different reasons. This idea was first proposed by Kurt Goldstein a century ago, in his article 'Das Symptom' (Goldstein, 1926). Later, it was more fully developed by Luria in his series of studies with soldiers that had penetrating brain injuries (most famously in World War II). Luria defined the 'qualitative' analysis of the syndrome as the 'study of the structure of the disturbance, and ultimately, by the identification of the factor or primary defect responsible for the development of the observable phenomenon' (Luria, 1980, p. 86). In the case of Sion, for example, his disinhibition might alter performance on *any* task, verbal or spatial. But his visuo-spatial problems form a quite different, and also *primary*, deficit.

Later in the last century, Edith Kaplan incorporated some of these ideas, formalising what today is known as the Process Approach to neuropsychological assessment (Kaplan, 1988a, 1988b; Libon et al., 2013). The origins of this way of thinking were actually far wider than Kaplan, and were unquestionably international. It included well-known figures such as the omni-present Aleksandr Luria (in the then USSR), Murial Lezak (on the west coast of the USA), Brenda Milner (in Canada) and Oliver Zangwill (in the UK). Our gnomic colleague, Kevin Walsh, arrives a generation after these pioneers (setting up his programme in the 1970s), and is famously Australian: in keeping with the international theme of clinical neuropsychology.

For reasons that are now clear, this was the field's response to the then-predominant 'psychometric' approach, which focused on test scores – and whether the test had been passed. Kaplan (and that community in general) emphasised that most standardised tests (e.g. problem-solving) had a multifactorial nature, thus offering a common source of interpretation error. They reminded us that, in order to understand how a complex psychological process has been altered by injury, it may be necessary to modify test administration, or introduce additional tests, making it possible to parse out the many factors involved in the particular measure. This 'process' approach would require a careful description, a 'qualification', of the nature of the error, from an understanding of the process or means by which the solution to a problem is reached (Libon et al., 2013).

What a snake-pit I had stumbled into with my little pyramid error. It had begun with a simple mistake: thinking that all measures of executive function are created equal. And it had been compounded by the oldest error in the book: looking only at what you *expect* to see, noticing only what makes sense to your existing worldview: classic confirmation bias. In doing this, I had taken an 'any three out of five' approach to executive tests, and looked at a scan only for the frontal lobes. Worse, I had stumbled into the middle of the most important debate in the last century of clinical neuropsychology: is it more important *whether* the patient fails a test, or *how* they fail? On the plus side, I had at least made a mistake about something very important. And, as a trainee, I had been offered a chance to learn from it.

References

Goldstein, K. (1926). Das Symptom, seine Entstehung und Bedeutung für unsere Auffassung vom Bau und von der Funktion des Nervensystems. *Archiv für Psychiatrie, 76,* 84–108.

Kaplan, E. (1988a). A process approach to neuropsychological assessment. In T. Boll & B. Bryant (Eds.), *Clinical Neuropsychology and Brain Function: Research, Measurement and Practice* (pp. 143–155). Washington, DC: APA.

Kaplan, E. (1988b). The process approach to neuropsychological assessment. *Aphasiology, 2*(3–4), 309–311.

Libon, D. J., Swenson, R., & Ashendorf, L. (2013). Edith Kaplan and the Boston process approach: A tribute to an original thinker. In L. Ashendorf, R. Swenson, & D. Libon (Eds.), *The Boston Process Approach to Neuropsychological Assessment: A Practitioner's Guide.* New York: Oxford University Press.

Libon, D. J., Swenson, R., Ashendorf, L., Bauer, R. M., & Bowers, D. (2013). Edith Kaplan and the Boston process approach. *The Clinical Neuropsychologist, 27*(8), 1223–1233.

Luria, A. (1980). *Higher Cortical Functions in Man.* New York: Basic Books.

6 Cutting corners

Oliver Turnbull

'The difference between the right word and the almost right word is really a large matter – it's the difference between lightning and a lightning bug'.

—Mark Tawin

1. Situation

There are probably places where you train as a clinical neuropsychologist in 'optimal' circumstances, or what some might view as optimal circumstances: for example, seeing only a limited number of patients in a week, but each with an interesting and varied background of pathologies, having enough time to test each patient for several hours, having access to comprehensive notes and scans, after having had a chance to review these in advance of the assessment, and with your supervisor down the corridor when you need them. I didn't train in one of those settings, and on reflection, it's probably better for me that I was exposed to the environment that I was.

The principal features of my training were that I saw lots of patients, and many of them for only an hour or two, which by neuropsychological standards is not for very long. On the plus side, this meant that I got to see an enormous diversity of neuropsychological disorders (an issue discussed in the Blindsight chapter).

But there was another element of not being able to see patients for long that I think has important implications: that a brief testing process makes you focus on psychological *functions* and *behaviour*, rather than simply on tests. A related point is that a brief assessment process forces the examiner to try to link test performance (where you don't have much information) with material that you derive during the *history* – importantly, because history taking is an extremely rich source of information, at least potentially.

Perhaps I can give an example of this. How should one assess audio-verbal short-term memory[1]? The industry standard is the systematic delivery of the Digit Span sub-test of the WAIS. The WAIS Instruction manual is quite clear on how to achieve this: you start with two digits forward, tested twice, then move upwards to three, and so on. Provided the patient is passing at least one

DOI:10.4324/9781003300748-6

of the items, you finally terminate the assessment of forward span on perhaps six or seven digits.

You then proceed to digits *backwards*, using the same system. You probably can't manage this in much faster than 5 minutes, and I think that subtest often takes closer to 10 minutes with many patients, who can become distracted. And remember that the gods of rigorous assessment will descend on you if administer it in an atypical way – for very good reason. It's a strict rule of the WAIS assessment process that you administer the test in a systematic way because – as every Clinical Psychology trainee knows – it needs to be delivered in the same way to compare the performance of the patient with the general population. Only that way you can establish a reliable Scaled Score, and a reliable overall measure of intelligence. This is a point on which we all agree. If you want to talk about Scaled Scores, and overall WAIS performance, then it's really important to deliver Digit Span exactly as described in the manual.

Now, there is a faster way of establishing whether verbal short-term memory is intact. First, you can make a provisional judgement based on the history. Where is the known, or the likely, lesion site? Was the patient able to follow the conversation? Did they have difficulty understanding your more complicated sentences? We use audio-verbal short-term memory all the time when we hold a conversation, so in a sense you're assessing the patient *throughout* the history. So, what to do with WAIS Digit Span, when you have the justified impression that your patient has intact short-term memory, and the lesion site information to back this up? Do you really have to start at the bottom, with two digits? In another famous gnome, Walsh reminds us that 'the difficult subsumes the easy' (Walsh, 1992, p. 127). If you suspect that your patient is within normal limits for the psychological function, you could give them a forward span of (say) five or six numbers. This takes 10 seconds to deliver, not 10 minutes. And if your patient can repeat six digits forward, then it's a fairly safe bet that this class of short-term memory ability is intact, and you've just saved yourself minutes of assessment time.

Let's look at this problem through a related example. Imagine that you're faced with a patient with a known left temporo-parietal lesion. That is, of course, the classic lesion site for producing an audio-verbal short-term memory impairment. You have time limitations – perhaps minutes to take a history, and for your assessment. You're not assessing for some sort of medico-legal report, or in order to establish some overall measure of intelligence. In fact, you're not even assessing short-term memory because you wonder *whether* it's impaired. You *know* it's likely to be impaired, because you can already see that your patient has the sort of word-finding problems and dysfluency that always follow from that lesion site. Now, are you going to use your precious assessment minutes on a standardised administration, or take a guess on a forward span of three or four (i.e. worse than the normal population), try that, and move up or down, depending on whether the patient passes or not? It will take 60 seconds to discover that the patient has a forward span of 3, as you expected.

Here is another example. Perhaps your patient has a *recent* memory disorder, for example after hippocampal damage, and you want to check short-term memory, in order to ensure that it's intact. It's almost certainly normal, because this time there is no left temporo-parietal lesion site. On the one hand, the classic diagnosis of recent memory impairment involves a demonstration that immediate memory is intact. Again, the technically correct approach is to deliver WAIS Digit Span by the book. But there isn't enough time – not without dropping something else important from the list. So, are you going take a guess on a forward span of six, try that and move up or down? Again, it will take 60 seconds to discover that the patient has a forward span of 6, as you expected.

Based on this sort of logic, I felt that I was getting good at flexible assessment (Bauer, 2000). And not just for short-term memory. I felt that I could judge the recent memory performance of my patients, starting with how they were doing during the history. And I could do the same with executive function, and expressive language ability and so on. I was getting used to evaluating the various component parts of the mind as I took my history, and then I would often deliver my psychological tests at a higher-level, to see whether my estimate was right or not.

Here, I was a big fan of the Cookie Theft picture. Superficially, it seems a simple task: 'What's going on in this picture?' In reality, it's a very complicated task, and not just because it has some rather poor perspective drawing, and out-of-date sex-role stereotypes. To complete the task, the patient needs to scan around a very complex scene of line drawing objects (which tests high-level vision). Then they need to draw inferences about who is doing what, for which reasons (which tests high-level executive function). And finally, they need to describe this to the examiner, using a coherently described grammatical narrative (which tests, amongst other things, high-level language ability). Now, I would never use the Cookie Theft picture, on its own, to draw conclusions about vision, executive function or language impairment. But if you are short of time, and your patient can sail through Cookie Theft in an effective way, then it's safe to say that vision, executive function and language are probably intact. And so, I was often able to draw inferences about core psychological processes, based on a combination of an astute listening between the lines of the history, and a rather cursory assessment of complex psychological processes – and I was becoming increasingly confident about this.

One of my favourite definitions of tragedy is: 'hubris meets nemesis': over-confidence gets what it deserves. The case described in the following is my little assessment tragedy, and it follows from my unjustified confidence that I could always listen between the lines during the history, and then do some rapid assessment, to then confirm my marvellous insights. In retrospect, there had been a fair bit of over-confidence going on. I'd seen a lot of patients, I felt that I was able to draw a lot of conclusions from the history, I was able to test psychological function based on limited test materials, and I was increasingly growing in confidence. In a well-constructed narrative, this would be an ideal time for me to meet my nemesis!

2. Case

Adam was a man in late middle age, who came to us with the referral letter from the clinician at a nearby government hospital. The referral letter was worryingly brief: centrally, it was a question about Adam's return to work, which was as a delivery driver for a medium-sized company. At face value, this was an interesting question for neuropsychologist, and one where I felt I might be able to offer an opinion. The referral was to our service because that hospital didn't have a neuropsychologist. Indeed, it turned out that many aspects of Adam's case were based on 'things that people didn't have', and ways that I had to try to work around those limitations. Ours was a service operating with limited resources. Looking back, I think that we were, in a strange sort of way, quite proud of being able to manage things despite this. Indeed, one of us (RC) has co-authored an entire book on how to cope as a neuropsychologist under these circumstances (Coetzer & Balchin, 2014).

So, which sort of things did Adam lack, and how could I solve these problems? First, Adam lacked any medical notes. Perhaps, in the modern world of electronic notetaking, and universal Wi-Fi, this must seem like a quaint scene from a historical costume drama. But actually, it was a relatively common circumstance, in our sometimes chaotic and challenged service. However, one doesn't acquire over-confidence by accident, and I had a solution to this problem: which is of course that I would ask the patient. Their history was, most of the time, good enough to get an impression of the medical circumstances.

It took me seconds to realise that the solution would be ineffective today, because Adam didn't speak English! This wasn't uncommon in our out-patient clinic, especially when we had patients referred from the more provincial parts of the country. But no worry, I had a solution to this problem: a translator. Doing neuropsychology through translation is not something that I would recommend for light entertainment, but it can be done. And I suspect that in a modern world of international migration and travel, it's not going to become any less common. Or not until someone invents the Babel Fish that Douglas Adams (1979) so charmingly imagined in his *Hitchhiker's Guide*.

My default solution for emergency translation was not, of course, to phone some hospital translation service (as if such a wonder existed . . .). It was instead to ask any of the nursing staff whether they spoke the requisite language, and could spare a bit of time to translate for me. It took me minutes to establish that all of the nursing staff were engaged in more important medical matters. And I had an outpatient waiting list for the afternoon, so I had no time to be trawling any of the wards on the hospital looking for translators. Nor indeed any credibility with the nursing staff of other wards to be asking them to give up an hour of their time. But no matter, I was a man of action, and I realised that it was another easy solution to this problem: which was that Adam had been brought by his daughter, who of course could act as translator. Throw me a problem, and I would find a solution.

The next challenge was the referral letter. As discussed in the Chapter on 'No such thing as a neuropsychological test', the best referral letters give you two things. First, some account of the *nature* of the medical problem, ideally narrowed down as much as possible. Second, the letter asks a referral question, ideally narrowed down as much as possible. Thus: 'My patient has *this* pathological process, which was acquired at *this* time, has progressed in *that* way, and has impaired their ability to do *x or y or z*'. That is Phase 1 of the referral letter, the survey of the medical history. Phase 2 then asks the critical referral question, which can of course take many forms: 'Can you explain why the patient has this unexpected problem'? and 'Can you suggest some form of appropriate treatment'?

The problem with Adam's referral letter was that it was all phase 2, but no phase 1. There was a clear referral question (could he return to work?), but no good idea about the medical history to this point. It was potentially frustrating. But no matter: I would take the medical history, without the assistance of medical notes, from the patient, working through his daughter as translator. It would be heroic.

Adam's daughter seemed a nice enough woman, perhaps in her mid-20s. She was wearing some sort of uniform, suggesting that she had probably taken the afternoon off to bring her father to hospital. I worked through the usual start to my assessments: name, age, education, occupation, handedness. . . . His daughter answered all the questions herself, and with good English. Impressively, I was managing without translation.

3. Error

And so, to the heart of the issue, what had happened to her father? An accident, she said. What sort of accident, I asked: a car accident? She asked her father, who responded in the affirmative. I sought to press for the usual details: how long ago, was there loss of consciousness, retrograde amnesia, duration of post-traumatic amnesia, associated medical problems, etc.? But now we ran into some difficulties. She lived in a different city, his daughter said, she hadn't been there at the time, and so she had only second-hand information. Could she ask her father what he remembered? She asked, he responded, and the translated answer was that he didn't really have any information to add. Which was unfortunate, but perhaps in the nature of memory impairment? Alas, asking an amnesic what they remember, through a translator, isn't much of an interrogation strategy.

It was about as poor a history as I've ever collected. But I did establish, from her, that the event had happened about six months ago. She had heard about it from her sister. Were there other things I could discover? Had her father suffered from any serious medical problems before his accident? No, he had been in good health.

And now, what was the principal complaint? Not from her father – I knew enough about closed head injury to know that the family often had a much better take on what the main post-morbid changes were. And I knew in advance what the answer was likely to be, of course: patients with closed head injury tend to be some combination of dysexecutive, with a mixture of disinhibited, disorganised and the like. Adam's daughter offered me one of the possible answers I might have been expecting: he was confused, and not clear about things, and this had caused lots of problems at work. In fact, he'd been sent home within minutes of trying to return to work a few weeks ago.

It was all fitting together: closed head injury, probably of reasonable severity, with some dysexecutive features. Which elements were they? Well, Adam certainly didn't look very disinhibited, at least behaviourally. But from the start I had noticed some elements of interaction with his daughter that suggested some difficulties. Most of the time it was *her* who had answered the questions. But when I specifically asked that she might *ask* her father, there was a rather asymmetrical back and forth between the two of the two of them. Sometimes he would give a long answer, which she translated in a few words. On other occasions a short answer generated quite a lot of translation. And most importantly, she seemed frustrated with her father's answers. Perhaps, or presumably, because he was somehow being disinhibited or socially inappropriate in his responses to his daughter, all not answering her questions properly, in that disorganised way so common with dysexecutive patients? It was all fitting together.

Next would be the assessment, using some standardised tests. For each test, I would put the materials on the table. I would explain the rules of each to Adam's daughter. She translated the rules, and then Adam completed the test. The tests overall were a mixed bag. Several decades later, I especially remember the worst of them: Controlled Oral Word Association (the test we commonly described as 'FAS'). As many words as possible, in 60 seconds, starting with F, there were no names of products, people, places or countries. His daughter translated, and he responded. Was I allowed to administer FAS in another language? Probably not, I guessed, but I thought I'd try it anyway, and ask Adam's daughter whether they were proper words. But Adam, unlike any of my other patients, didn't respond with a list of words, but with what sounded like a sentence, where things didn't all start with F. I asked his daughter how it was going? He can't think of any words she said. Nothing? Not one word? It was still 45 seconds on my stopwatch. He was not good with words, she said. As I told you, he gets confused . . . I'd never written 'no words' down next to the letter F. We tried starting with the letter A, but of course it was no better. Zero. The worst Controlled Oral Word Association performance I'd ever seen.

Not all the measures of executive function were so catastrophically bad. He was quite a bit better on the Rey Complex Figure, where he produced a reasonable copy performance, and then a rather more modest drawing on recall. Frontal amnesia, I assumed, which of course he was entitled to. In retrospect, this pattern of dissociation between good performance on the visual spatial tasks of executive function, and frankly catastrophic performance on the verbal tasks, might have rung an alarm bell. But at the back of my mind was the recollection that the performance of dysexecutive patients on these sorts of tasks can be quite variable – good at some, poorer at others. And, in retrospect, I might have listened a little harder to his daughter's repeated observations but he 'wasn't good with words', and that he 'got confused'.

But all of that didn't make any difference, because the case was done and dusted. Adam had had a head injury, presumably a rather serious one; of course we were in no position to confirm that. His daughter had complained that he had difficulty with various complicated things, his employer had sent him home on his first day of return to work, yet been inappropriate in his conversations with his daughter, and had done catastrophically badly on several of my measures of executive function.

It was going to be a reasonably easy letter to write back to the referrer. Yes, he was dysexecutive. Luckily, he was in a job which could be reasonably well managed if it were highly structured. Perhaps if things could be re-organised so that the level of complex decision-making in his role was minimised, things might be fine.

On the way out of the assessment room, I ran into one of the neurology Registrars. Drawing together two parallel strands of my life, I realised that they spoke the same language as Adam. Perhaps they were in a better position to ask Adam's daughter to ask about the duration of post-traumatic amnesia? Could the Registrar spare five minutes to chat to Adam and try to complete the history? Sure, they could find a few minutes. I stood to one side while Adam and the Registrar had a chat. And every once in a while, the Registrar looked back at me, with an increasing sense of surprise. He then asked Adam and his daughter to sit down for a few minutes, while we had a chat separately. Are you *sure* he's had a head injury, the Registrar said? That's what his daughter told me, she told me he'd had an accident? Interesting, the Registrar said. And what about his language, you do know he doesn't understand a thing? My jaw dropped. What did the Registrar mean? His language comprehension is terrible, she said. And he produces nothing but word salad . . . absolute nonsense. I'd guess it's Wernicke's, the Registrar suggested, delicately. Why would you get that from a head injury? It was a long pause. And then I said . . . because he hasn't *had* a head injury . . . because what his daughter called an 'accident', was a stroke? And because I've been an idiot.

In some sort of dissociated state, the assessment flashed before my eyes. His doctor said he'd had an accident . . . his employer knew within minutes that he couldn't return to work . . . his daughter kept telling me that he wasn't good at understanding words . . . and his word fluency was zero but his visual spatial performances weren't too bad. And all because I thought that I could manage without proper medical history, and without a proper translator. And because I was a complete idiot.

Over the next few weeks, I was prone to flashbacks of the trauma of it all. One of the most recurrent thoughts was that I'd been unlucky to get 'the wrong aphasia'. What if Adam had had some sort of expressive aphasia, like the classic Broca's? There was no way that I would have missed that – because it's not that difficult to identify hesitant speech, and word-finding difficulty, even in a foreign language. And patients with expressive aphasia almost always have some sort of right-sided weakness. If Adam had presented with non-fluent speech, and a right hemiplegia, I would never have fallen for the argument that he had a closed head injury. Mind you, I wouldn't have made the mistake if I hadn't been assessing through his daughter as a translator. Or indeed if I'd had access to the medical notes, or asked the referring clinician for better detail in their referral letter. But you can't run a life on 'what ifs', and the simple truth was that I had cut too many corners.

I made my excuses to the Registrar. And I told Adam's daughter that I needed to get back and assess her father again. But only at *next* week's out-patient appointment, once I'd had a chance to get the medical records, and contact the doctor at the other hospital that had referred him, so that had a better understanding of her father's medical history. At next time, I would arrange for a translator that I trusted.

4. Reflection

There are several clear elements that conspired to create this embarrassing problem. At the heart of it lies the over-confidence that I could cut all sorts of corners, and still deliver a reasonable assessment. With the wisdom of hindsight, I would say that there *might* be times when you can cut some corners. There are also clear times when you would not want to cut corners: a forensic setting might be top of the list, but I could think of many others. So, choose your times wisely, try not to cut too many, and for heaven's sake be careful not to cut too deep.

What of the specific problems? Clearly having the medical notes would have solved the key problem in a moment. Yes, you can get a history from the patient, or indeed from the patient's family. But there so many things that are best mediated by other members of the medical profession. This problem needed a better referral letter, and access to the medical notes. Or at very least, one of the two? Clearly, there are exceptional circumstances in which medical notes or a referral is not available. And clearly the advice would be to proceed with caution, and an awareness of how you are limiting yourself.

In addition, working with translators is difficult, but it is clearly better if the translator is someone who is neutral to the situation, and ideally is someone with some medical knowledge. Family members or friends have a worrying habit of giving you *their* version of the patient's story. I would be especially aware if the length of the translation doesn't match the patient's answer. The stereotype is a one-minute answer from the patient, to which the translator reports: 'The patient says yes'. You want to know what the patient said, not what the translator has filtered. I would also try and ask short, factual sentences, such as 'When was the accident?', or 'Do you sometimes get lost when walking around town?', where there is less room for interpretation. Avoid open-ended questions, such as 'Tell me about your accident'. These generate long answers, with lots of opportunity for the translator to add their spin to the story. At very least, I should not have accepted his daughter's *summary* of her father's answers. Instead, I should have asked for what he said *exactly*, word for word.

And finally, there is the assessment of executive function. It's true that there is often variability in performance between tests of executive ability. But there is one general principle that I think offers clarity: that test failure should broadly match psychological processes, on all possible fronts. Thus: is the patient failing on all (or most of) the tests of disinhibition, and do they fail them in a way that *looks* qualitatively disinhibited, and does this match the account of everyday behaviour reported by the family, and is the patient disinhibited during the history-taking and assessment? Adam's pattern of executive payment wasn't consistent in this way at all – there wasn't a narrative of *one* impaired psychological process. There were vast differences between scores, but no pattern across function. That absence should have rung alarm bells.

In brief, there were lots of reasons for me to be worried about Adam's case, and they followed from cutting far too many corners, without an awareness of the risks I was taking. That doesn't mean that I couldn't cut corners. However, with apologies to Abraham Lincoln, you can't cut all of the corners all of the time. At best, you might allow yourself to cut *some* of the corners some of the time – and with caution.

Note

1 Sometimes (arguably) called immediate memory, which is probably identical with the phonological loop component of working memory, and so on. All too often, there are several terms for one process in neuropsychology. On the positive side, knowing that many terms can refer to a single process can make the trainee's life a lot simpler.

References

Adams, D. (1979). *The Hitchhiker's Guide to the Galaxy*. London: Ballantine Books.
Bauer, R. (2000). The flexible battery approach to neuropsychological assessment. In R. Vanderploeg (ed.) *Clinical Guide to Neuropsychological Assessment* (pp. 419–448). New York: Routledge.
Coetzer, R. & Balchin, R. (2014). *Working With Brain Injury: A Primer for Psychologists Working in Under-Resourced Settings*. London: Psychology Press.
Walsh, K. (1992). Some gnomes worth knowing. *Clinical Neuropsychologist*, 6(2), 119–133. https://doi.org/10.1080/13854049208401849

7 Blind sight

Oliver Turnbull

'That they behold, and see not what they see?'

—William Shakespeare

1. Situation

With increasing experience as a trainee, it's easy to become more interested in the 'seaside zoo' approach to neuropsychology. By this, we mean the idea that (like any aspirational zoo) you have to have an example of every species on the premises, which is how I was beginning to feel about neuropsychological disorders. I was learning so much from seeing neurological patients. It was one thing to get the description of patients in textbooks. However, it is another thing entirely to meet the patients in person. Whenever I encountered a real-life example of someone with a neuropsychological disorder, I thought that I would know the presentation for ever. The problem, of course, was seeing all the various neuropsychological disorders. The world is, I discovered, full of dysexecutive patients, of patients with hemispatial neglect, of patients with expressive, agrammatical aphasia. But who wants to see the same disorder over and over again, I thought? And so, I became increasingly interested in the rare, in the exotic.

In my most obsessional phase, I started to make lists, based on the categories of neuropsychological disorder described in my favourite textbooks. There were, I thought, probably six, seven or eight categories of aphasia. One might debate whether the 'receptive' variant was called Wernicke's aphasia or a loss of auditory comprehension. But that was clearly one 'kind'. And the variant had intact comprehension, but poor repetition. . . . Well, that used to be called conduction aphasia, and Luria called it acoustic-amnestic aphasia, and the cognitive neuropsychologists might call it an audio-verbal short-term memory problem. But they were all clearly type number two. And so, I had my list of six, seven or eight categories of acquired language impairment.

But, of course, it doesn't end with aphasia. There were all of the various kinds of amnesia, and all the alexias, the agraphias, the apraxias and so on – three, five and seven types in each category. So there I was, like some sort of neuropsychological stamp collector, seeing whether I could encounter at least

DOI:10.4324/9781003300748-7

one of each category. It was a fairly obsessional worldview, but I was making progress with seeing examples of lots of them. I'd seen five of the six types of aphasia (I was missing a transcortical motor aphasia), almost all of the acalculias (but no primary anarithmetria), and I was missing a good case of ideational apraxia. But I was doing well.

However, in all of this, there was a big gap surrounding the agnosias. These are, of course, well-known disorders in neuropsychology – famous historically. They were the foundation of our understanding of higher vision, and had been described by Lissauer an age ago (1890). The stamp collecting side of me knew that there were two principal kinds. But the realist was also beginning to understand that they were extremely rare. And so it was with some interest that I received a referral from one of our rehabilitation units on the other side of town. Indeed, from a unit distinctly on the wrong side of the tracks. But the occupational therapist was very clear: she had a patient who *could* see, but *couldn't* see. He'd been in an accident at work, and now he was 'blind'. Except that he wasn't blind. Just like the classical descriptions. When I received the telephone call, she might as well have just told me that she'd discovered a unicorn!

2. Example

James was a man in his 40s, who had worked in the building trade, at the manual labour end of the work spectrum. He was a nice enough man, happy enough to give me a clear history – which was uneventful, until his industrial accident, where he'd been exposed to some nasty chemicals, while cleaning out a large container. They'd found him, collapsed and unconscious, on the floor. But he'd made a good general medical recovery, and was able to stand and walk, understand and talk, and indeed hold a reasonable conversation with me. To be honest, you'd be hard pressed to know he was a neurological patient on meeting him, were it not that there was no eye contact. He looked *at* me, or at least he looked roughly in the direction of my face, but he seemed to look through me. As the minutes passed, I realised that this was because he wasn't really fixating on parts of my face. I hadn't thought about it before, but people's eyes were always darting across my face – looking at my eyes and mouth, perhaps glancing at my hands, but always moving, and that movement was a sign of their attention.

So, did James have that 'thousand-yard stare' first coined during the World Wars? Was he looking blankly forward, staring 'through' me? No. Actually, his eyes were quite *active*. But, as time went by, I realised that they weren't stopping on the various important parts of my face – or indeed even at my face at all. He was just darting his eyes around in the general direction of my voice. There was eye *movement*, but there wasn't eye *contact*. Also, there was a 'modality' issue here too. I'd never met one of those 'thousand-yard stare' characters, by which I presume they meant soldiers traumatised by the immediate experience of war and death. But I was prepared to bet that the soldiers' voices were consistent with their eye movements – all long pauses and dark answers. But James was a man of mixed modality messages: no contact through the eyes, while holding a lively conversation with his voice.

But that was enough of the history. And by now, I could see that most of the important bits of cognition were probably intact. He always understood me, and his speech was fluent and anomia-free. And his turn-taking abilities in language, his coherent account of his history, and his appropriate answers to my questions all suggested at least reasonable executive function. I just needed to check some posterior brain areas.

I decided to start with some low-level vision. Normally, I would investigate both hemi-fields, and to see what his visual acuity was. With James it was perhaps more a question of whether he had any visual field at all? After a few seconds of assessment, some general principles became clear. First, he didn't seem able to respond to *all* to my wiggling fingers. I'd seen patients with neglect, who were fine in one hemi-field, and blind in the other. But this was different. James was able to respond my wiggles just *some* of the time. Indeed, after some trial and error, it seemed that he would be much better if I made more substantial movements. So, he wasn't blind, and (unlike neglect) there was no laterality effect, or at least none that I could see.

The next matter would be to progress with the quality issue. How many fingers was I holding up? Which of my fingers was I showing him? How many dots were there on this piece of paper? Here he was quite prepared to take a guess at numbers, but I didn't think that he was doing much better than chance. He could see *something*, but it wasn't entirely clear *what* he could see. I tried to get some impression of his subjective experience in all of this. What did he 'see'? Could he see me? Yes, he could, he told me. But things were sometimes a bit blurry. Blurry? That seemed an understatement!

Next, I wanted to get some idea about object recognition. Most neuropsychologists have a test for that in their bag of tricks, and it usually doubles as a naming test, of the sort that is helpful in assessing aphasia. I pulled out my naming test out and showed him the pictures. He was terrible at the task, though it was interesting to see the way that he had at least *some* knowledge. For example, he would often say 'it's some kind of animal'. And he was sometimes right about that. He would then take a guess: 'It's a cow' or 'It's a pig'. On the specifics, he was almost invariably wrong, or at least not much better than guessing at whatever chance level was. For the pictures of inanimate objects, he was again able to make some sort of broad category judgement. 'Some kind of big thing' he suggested, to the picture of a lorry, presumably because it was chunky? And 'some kind of little thing' to picture of a pen. Which he guessed was a stick.

But I wasn't done with object recognition. Like any good trainee, I was capable of sometimes being a day ahead of the game in knowledge. I'd known that James might have visual agnosia, so I'd searched through the relevant chapter of a few textbooks, and discovered some important things. One of them was that the quality of object recognition depended on the nature of the stimulus. Apparently, recognition of line drawings was the poorest, things were better with photographs, especially colour photographs, and things were best with real objects. One chapter on the topic had been particularly enlightening, because it had explained why this effect existed. It had to do with the number of visual cues available from each format. Line drawings had very few sources of information: all two-dimensional, with no sense of contours, nor of colour, nor of texture. Upgrade to a photograph, and you had a better sense of contour, and colour, and of whether the texture was furry, or shiny, or scaly. But it was still two-dimensional, and there was no sense of scale either, because both an elephant and a mouse can be the same size in a photograph. With a real object you got all of the above, and the added advantage that you could view the object from several perspectives. That seemed to explain the difference.

So, what had I brought in my bag of tricks? A good experimentalist would have had a set of colour and black and white photographs, matched to the line drawings that I'd showed James in the object naming task a few minutes earlier. No chance of that. Indeed, I'm not sure that such a matched set of those stimuli existed back then. So the next time, I saw him I improvised, with some pictures from magazines and children's books. What did James think of these? He still struggled, but seemed to do a little better. In fact, he seemed to use the colour and texture information quite well, together with clues from body parts. He got the pig correct, muttering something about the snout, and probably helped by the pinkness and the curly tail? But one could also see how this piecemeal approach could be a problem. He was quite confident that one picture was a horse: 'You can see it from the brown coat', he said. Except that it was a kangaroo!

So, I knew some very important things, which meant that he really did have a visual agnosia. First, James wasn't blind. As with so many neuropsychological disorders, you need to demonstrate at least some degree of intact primary sensory capability before you can talk about impairment in the perceptual and synthetic ability. You can't have Wernicke's aphasia if you're deaf. And you can't have visual agnosia if you're blind. Second, James had the core impairment visual agnosia: the failure of object recognition. This 'filling' in the diagnostic sandwich: despite some degree of intact sensation, he had great difficulty using this visual knowledge. He couldn't count the number of things, and he couldn't recognise objects. The third element was that his impairment should not be a result of a more generalised cognitive disorder. You can't have an agnosia, for example, if you have dementia. And it should be modality-specific: other sense modalities, like hearing and tactile sensation, should be intact. Luckily, James clearly had many other areas of intact cognitive function: we had held a conversation, he had understood what I was saying, he spoke fluently, he remembered of the parts of a conversation, and cross-referenced. This was no dementia. And most importantly it appeared to be a modality specific problem: he could recognise things through the auditory modality (my voice), but apparently not through vision.

And finally, I needed to deliver on the most interesting and important test that I could for a patient with visual agnosia: I need to get him to copy a line drawing. Obviously, I wouldn't be expecting him to *recognise* the object – I'd assessed that earlier, and James was very poor at recognising line drawings. But how might we expect his *copying* to look? On the one hand, you might expect it to be really terrible. After all he was, apparently, some variant of 'blind'? Surely if you can't recognise an object, that would be because you couldn't 'see' it properly, and then you couldn't copy it either. On the other hand, it would be the most remarkable paradox if someone were able to copy line drawings, but not to be able to recognise them? The patient would be in a strange situation in which they could use visual knowledge for *one* thing (copying) but not *another* (recognising). So, which category could a patient with visual agnosia belong to?

I had been working away in my text books the previous night, and had discovered that the answer was, one way or another: both! That is, there were some patients who couldn't recognise, and *couldn't* copy either and others who couldn't recognise, but yet *could* copy. This was an old distinction, dating all the way back to Lissauer. Like all high-quality neuropsychological disorders, the distinction even came with a fancy bit of etymology of Greek and Latin origin. Some patients, it seemed, had more low-level impairments of vision, and could neither copy nor recognise. Lissauer had called this 'apperceptive' agnosia, because they were somehow disorders of perception. They reflected an inability to build a stable model of the shape of objects. Understandably, their ability to copy was terrible, and often involved failure to understand even spatial fundamentals like the orientation of lines, or the relative location of objects (or part-objects). They weren't blind, but their vision was no more accurate than someone looking through a kaleidoscope. Other patients showed that remarkable dissociation between equally poor object recognition but an *intact* ability to copy. Lissauer had called this 'associative' agnosia. It was associative, in that the basic perceptual mechanisms seemed intact, but there were difficulties linking (or associating) these to the world of concepts (which one would presumably need for recognition?). Which was James to be?

I brought along a reasonably complex line for James to copy, and gave him a blank piece of paper and a pencil to work from. I only wish I still had a copy of his original artwork, but alas it's lost now. However, a few years later, while I was completing my PhD, I found another of these rare neurological patients (DM), and investigated him in much more detail. We published a paper based on it (Turnbull et al., 2004), and I've reproduced the copying performance of the patient here (see Figure 7.1).

DM's performance shows the same sort of copy and characteristics that James showed, in the context of a similar sort of visual agnosia. It's a performance of remarkable detail and accuracy, in parts – including the cap, the face and some elements of the shirt and trousers, with lots of highly specific detail. In some respects, as good a performance as some neurologically normal people might manage. But that's only true for about 90% of the drawing. There are some really striking errors. Notably, they are at the clearest when it comes to the junction *between* object-parts, when one component is hidden behind another. For example, in the original, the right hand wraps around the cone. But DM

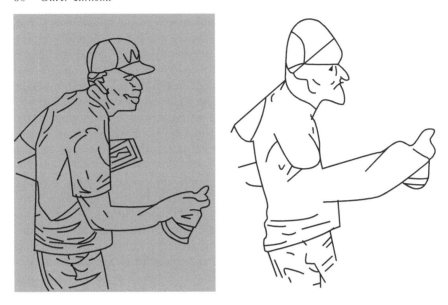

Figure 7.1 DM's copy of a figure, including failures to separate 3D object parts from the 2D image.

copies the hand and ice cream cone as if he doesn't really understand they are two separate objects? Or the way that the right upper arm fits into the right sleeve? It's not clear that he has understood the 'arm' and 'sleeve' concepts. It's as if DM sees many of the individual lines very accurately, but they aren't much more than lines – so that they don't form themselves into coherent objects. In some respects, DM sees the world with a fair amount of visual accuracy, but little visual meaning. This is perhaps the same way that we can all repeat – or almost repeat – a phrase in a foreign language, without having any understanding of auditory meaning.

So, now that I knew he had an agnosia, and that the cause was some sort of problem broadly localised to the posterior circulation. As with all good neuropsychological assessment, I could investigate other likely phenomena from that vascular territory. One obvious candidate was his recent memory. I knew that the posterior circulation placed the hippocampus at high risk. But he had seemed not to be memory impaired when I took the history, and even a fairly brief formal investigation suggested that his recent memory seemed very less intact. Or at least that it was intact for verbal material. Given his visuo–spatial impairments, it would have been inappropriate to test recent memory using a medium that we knew he was impaired on (an issue discussed in Chapter 5).

Then I was in a position to try and investigate a few other phenomena of the posterior brain. I didn't have a lot of time to do this, and I certainly didn't have the sorts of sophisticated test materials that I might have needed. But

I did my best to try and tick off a few other disorders with fancy names. Did he have prosopagnosia? Yes, in the sense that he couldn't recognise faces. But, of course, his low level visual abilities were worryingly modest anyway, so I'm not sure I could merit giving him the specific diagnosis? Similarly with reading. He clearly couldn't read, but I'm not sure that I'd have said that he had a specific alexia (rather than a reading failure due to poor basic perceptual abilities). Was he simultanagnosic? Probably not, in that he didn't seem to fixate, and become locked on, a specific object in his visual field. Finally, I was a little more confident that he had some form of achromatopsia. Though I had to test this by pointing at coloured objects, and I couldn't always be sure that he was judging the same object that I was pointing to. But, one way or another, I would certainly have a long list of fancy sounding names to recite off when I was describing the case.

In retrospect, James also had an area of preservation which was important, but which I hadn't really noticed. Or at least I hadn't paid enough attention to. This was the fact that his ability to use vision to reach out and grab things, for example a mug on a table, was intact. Or I vaguely remember it being intact. Or I at least don't remember him being clumsy? Usually called 'visually guided action' these days, I'm embarrassed to report that I wasn't really aware of it then. In retrospect, I probably didn't notice it because the important scientific literature on the topic hadn't yet been published when I was training. This was the famous 'two cortical visual systems' account, best known now from the work of David Milner and Mel Goodale (Goodale & Milner, 1992; Goodale et al., 1992; Milner & Goodale, 1995). The core of this work is another patient, DF, in whom recognition is hugely impaired (i.e. she has visually agnosia like James), but for whom reaching and grasping were entirely preserved. In my recollection, James would also have showed this dissociation too. I've noticed this a lot over the years with neuropsychological disorders. It's amazing how, once someone *else* describes a new phenomenon, you realise that you had previously assessed a patient with that pattern of impaired and intact ability. But, of course, I lacked the theoretical framework to understand that at the time. It makes me wonder how many other disorders there are that other scientists and clinicians have yet to reveal?

Regardless of this, my assessment had wound to its (apparently successful?) conclusion. My patient had a core diagnosis, and that diagnosis was associative visual agnosia. And I had a nice list of other disorders to discuss too: prosopagnosia, alexia, simultanagnosia and achromatopsia. Especially enjoyable if one was interested in fancy Greek technical terms. The diagnostic work was more or less done, and I was able to return to the therapist who had referred James and report my findings. However, as I was recounting things to her, I realised that my diagnostic acumen was actually far from a triumph. She had, after all, contacted me saying that she thought the patient *had* a visual agnosia. All of my assessment had merely been to confirm that fact, and indeed to add a small element of detail: to add the label 'associative', and throw in a few extra bits of terminology.

3. Error

Putting it that way made it seem much less of a diagnostic success. Indeed, it rather left me wondering whether I was just continuing with my 'stamp collecting', or whether I was going to add some clinical value to the case. And then the therapist offered me the opportunity to do just that. She had been thinking about an intervention, she said, and she was aware that there was a local centre which offered retraining for the blind. Did I think that this might be helpful for James? I didn't have much time to think about it, but it seemed reasonably clear to me that he should be able to make quite good gains. After all, I pointed out, James had *more* vision than those with peripheral blindness had! And so James was referred to a different part of the medical system, where he would receive training along with patients who had glaucoma, diabetic retinopathy, and macular degeneration.

I didn't hear of James for several months, until I returned again to the hospital, to see a completely different case. I popped into the therapy rooms to see how things had gone. Unfortunately, the news wasn't good. James had attended the course, and all the way through. But he had made disturbingly little progress, and their clinical lead had contacted my therapist, to enquire as to why he had done so badly. Why had we referred on a patient who had made so little gain? And besides, he wasn't really blind, and other clinician had pointed out. All in all, the referral had created a bit of a problem.

I was stunned. After all the logic behind my argument had seemed obvious. And so I took the problem to my clinical supervisor. Alas, in our discussion, a great deal more became clear. The mechanism of treatment for the peripherally blind (people with problems in the orbit itself, like diabetic retinopathy and macular degeneration) follows the rehabilitation argument outlined so clearly in neuropsychology by Alexander Luria. Here, the goal is to replace *one* failing sensory modality with one that is intact. The blind may have lost *vision*, but they can use other senses to build up an accurate model of the world. For example, when it comes to dealing with objects close to them (in peri-personal space, we might say) they can use touch to inform their spatial awareness. I can feel that this object is shaped like *this*, and by touch (and perhaps also by sound) I know is located *there*. To rephrase the argument, an intact central system (visuo-spatial ability) is now informed by a different sensory modality (touch instead of vision). The task for the blind individual is to practice with the new modality, to build up experience and a sense of control. But as both the sense of touch and the brain's visuo-spatial ability are intact, this is eminently achievable.

However, the problem James faced was that there was *no* intact central system: the impairment was to the central spatial system in the first place! Indeed, my supervisor reminded me, we saw exactly the same issue in patients with aphasia. For example, in the classical expressive aphasias (what we might call expressive or Broca's aphasia), we see a *spoken* language production which is agrammatical, principally through a lack of function words (words like: and, if, then, how, etc.) and also through difficulty accessing verbs and adjectives. The beginner neuropsychologist might imagine that the patient should therefore be able to communicate normally using *writing*. After all, language production using the hand is a different output channel to that of using the muscles of articulation. But the lesson from 150 years of the aphasiology is that these patients tend to show similar sorts of language production whether it is through spoken language *or* written language. The impairment in these cases is one of the *central* mechanisms that controls language, so that it makes no difference which output modality they use. James was a perceptual equivalent of the same problem. Because he had lost the central spatial mechanism, it made no difference which sensory system was used to access this. And hence the programme for the blind had been doomed to failure.

It was a shattering moment of realisation. In one example, I was able to see the key difference between core psychological processes, and the more specialised peripheral sensory and motor systems which they used. My supervisor then sent me to reread the final chapters of the Luria's (1973) famous book *The Working Brain*. I'd read it before, and I'd been impressed by the way in which he managed to synthesise complex functional systems (for language, perception, problem-solving, etc.), putting together a range of basic skills in the service of much more complex psychological processes. Now, with my changed perspective on the role of a peripheral versus central abilities, I viewed the chapters in a new light.

4. Reflection

On my third visit to the hospital, I returned to speak to my therapist colleague. I explained to her that I had finally understood why James wasn't able to make the gains from treatment that the programme for the blind offered. Why he was in many respects in an even worse position than someone who was blind to make such gains. And I apologised for offering such poor advice.

Today, thinking about this story, I wonder what the lessons are to be learned. Perhaps the most important one is that neuropsychological assessment is not simply a *diagnostic* endeavour. From the patient's standpoint, it is a tool to gather information that can be helpful in planning *how* to manage deficits and reduce their impact in everyday life. In other words, patients don't expose themselves to long and painful hours of testing just to learn that their problem has a specific name which derives from some strange Greek word. They come to us because they hope we can help them understand what is going on, and to help manage the problem. The same principle can be applied to assessment referrals from colleagues. Good neuropsychological assessment should be inseparable from rehabilitation. This might seem obvious, but it is not, particularly because the knowledge about how the brain relates to basic and complex psychological processes (i.e. neuropsychology) is not the same as the knowledge for *rehabilitating* those processes when damaged. Clinical neuropsychologists must become familiar with *both* languages, and learn how to translate ideas from one to the other. To return to the analogy with which this chapter began, we should never forget that the 'seaside zoo' approach to neuropsychology is useful in acquiring knowledge of the many species we must learn to differentiate. However, our main task is to help to *care* for the species.

Good clinical neuropsychologists can learn from their mistakes. Indeed, they have to. I hadn't been able to help my patient very much at all. However, he had unquestionably helped me. It's a simple, and perhaps over-used, line of argument: to talk about how clinicians learn so much from their patients. But that doesn't mean that it's not true. And it's especially true in the neurological sciences, where the problems are so complex, where there is so much that we still don't know, and where treatments are currently all too rare, and all too modest in their effects. It's a disturbing thought that we might wake up in the morning with a desire to help our patients, but go to bed at night with the realisation that they have helped us.

References

Goodale, M.A. & Milner, A.D. (1992). Separate visual pathways for perception and action. *Trends in Neuroscience*, *15*(1): 20–25.

Goodale, M.A., Milner, D.A., Jakobson, L.S. & Carey, D.P. (1992). A neurological dissociation between perceiving objects and grasping them. *Nature*, *349*: 154–156.

Lissauer, H. (1890). Ein Fall von Seelenblinheit nebst einem Beitrag zur Theorie derselben. *Archiv für Psychiatrie*, *21*: 222–270.

Luria, A.R. (1973). *The working brain*. Aylesbury: Penguin.

Milner, A.D. & Goodale, M.A. (1995) *The visual brain in action*. Oxford: Oxford University Press.

Turnbull, O.H., Driver, J. & McCarthy, R.A. (2004). 2D but not 3D: Pictorial-depth deficits in a case of visual agnosia. *Cortex*, *40*: 723–738.

8   I did it my way

Rudi Coetzer

'It would be wise to remember that the law of parsimony has never been repealed'.
—Walsh (1992) *Some gnomes worth knowing*

1. Situation

Clinical neuropsychologists apparently come in two versions. Some are disparingingly referred to as 'touchy feely', who are much more focused on rehabilitation and psychological therapy. And then there are the 'testers', or psycho-diagnosticians. Listening to colleagues, one is often led to believe that each side tends to view their role as the more important. A similar distinction is the dualistic 'practitioner-academic' conceptualisation. An oxymoron if ever there was one, as any clinical neuropsychologist worth their salt needs to be up to date both academically and practically. It's really just about bias, and the distinction is not even that static, as clinicians may become more or less academically active with time.

To return to the point that some colleagues view diagnostics and rehabilitation to be diametrically opposed, this is of course an illogical way to reason about the core skills of the profession. Perhaps, rather than 'sub-specialities', within clinical neuropsychology, this erroneous view actually confuses the concepts of employment, and daily work. Where we are employed, at least to some degree, may influence our subjective professional identity, but it does not change our actual profession. Like many things, it is about the balance between these two ingredients, rather than the absolutes. Me? I'm definitely in the 'touchy-feely' camp, having served my 'test donkey' years, in a major university medical school teaching hospital. These seem ample experience to prove I can test as well as any of my colleagues in the other camp.

2. Example

Time ceased to function when I saw David. He was a stockily built man in his early 20s, with an expressionless face. When looking at David, the only defining visual feature seemed to me to be his spectacles. The lenses to correct his myopia were so powerful; it distorted his eyes to look almost artificial. They

DOI:10.4324/9781003300748-8

were asymmetrical to the rest of his face, as one would see through a camera with a fish-eye lens.

Other than that, there was little to remember him by, other than the question of speed. You see, David was so slow in his performance of cognitive tasks, in fact *any* tasks, that time seemed to me to freeze solid. My first encounter with him was his neuropsychological assessment, before I could become involved in the (for me) more interesting part of his care, rehabilitation. Testing over five sessions. More of that later. First, a background history had to be completed.

David's history was as follows. He sustained a traumatic brain injury when he was run over by a car approximately two years earlier. David was part of a group of people walking next to the road, when hit by a drunk driver. One person died, and David sustained a head injury. There was no mention of other injuries in the ambulance staff's notes, except some minor abrasions to his arms. In fact, the hospital medical notes were also rather sparse, containing very little other than his daily observations. He spent one week in hospital, before being discharged home. David has been unable to return to his work as a tyre fitter since the accident. He lived with his parents, which was apparently the same situation as before the injury. David reported no problems at school, and told me he obtained the equivalent of two A level qualifications, in History and English.

Obtaining a more complete history from David was very difficult, to say the least. He was just so vague and slow, that it was very laborious to try and cover all the relevant aspects of his history. It took a considerable amount of time just to obtain the basics. David did not think he had any problems prior to the accident. He had no previous surgery or illnesses of note, and had never required any input from a mental health team. Returning to his head injury, what did transpire was that he could not remember a thing about being run over, nor for at least a week prior to the accident. And he had no memory for weeks afterwards. In fact, he appeared having ongoing memory problems – forgetting things from one week to the other during our assessment appointments. There was growing evidence that David had sustained a severe traumatic brain injury: a large retrograde amnesia, and indeed post-traumatic amnesia, and the referrer comments of a clinical diagnosis of diffuse axonal injury.

David was referred to our service with a request for neuropsychological and neuropsychiatric assessment, and thereafter rehabilitation. The neuropsychiatric assessment was presumably to determine if he was depressed, or presenting with severe apathy secondary to a traumatic brain injury. Our first session was fully taken up with obtaining that brief history. During the second consultation, a clinical assessment was completed, including bedside cognitive testing, and a mental status examination.

With prompting and encouragement, David appeared to be able to demonstrate a rough orientation for time and place. But other bedside tests, such as reverse counting and reverse spelling, to assess concentration, struck a blank. He seemed quite unable to do these fairly simple tasks – the same for new learning and retention. It was like trying to draw blood from an immovable granite stone. It seemed David could not retain any facts. Tests of executive function were also too difficult for him, and at times it looked almost as if he did not comprehend what was required of him during a task, despite several attempts at explaining what was required of him.

Mental status examination again clearly illustrated David's main problems: he was really slow, and just did not initiate spontaneous conversation. And it wasn't just that his speech itself was slow. The time taken to respond to questions was excruciatingly lengthy. This opened up other avenues. Was he possibly depressed? This seemed less likely. It was true that he expressed little or no positive affect. But verbally he did retain a robust sense of future. He also reported sleeping well, and that his appetite was very good. Indeed to the extent that he had gained weight. His sense of smell and taste was preserved to, and did not seem to have interfered with his enjoyment of food. There were no symptoms of anxiety. In summary, David's thought processes and perceptual functions were in many respects entirely normal. However, his slowness, poor memory and lack of initiation, might fit with a history of severe traumatic brain injury. Formal neuropsychological testing was now the next step in David's assessment.

Neuropsychological testing took much, much longer than anticipated, even factoring in David's slowness. I regularly caught myself silently cursing that testing David was such a waste of time. I should be trying to help this unfortunate man. For heaven's sake, he sustained a severe traumatic brain injury, with diffuse axonal injury. It's a purely academic exercise to add numbers and percentiles, and it's not adding to what seemed painfully obvious in the consultation room. Diagnostic neuropsychology could be, I thought, as dull as tepid dishwater. Maybe I should ask the assistant psychologist to do the testing. Actually, that would be a bad idea, I decided, and continued testing him.

Why? Because David and I had already developed a good rapport, and this would be helpful for when I started the therapeutic work he will undoubtedly require. Without a robust therapeutic relationship, David would be less likely to buy into the rehabilitation strategies I had in mind – to help reduce the impact of his poor memory on his daily life. For now, though, formal testing had to be completed, and scored. This was fairly pointless, alas, as I was already sure that his results would only confirm the obvious impairments from his traumatic brain injury.

David's psychometric results were clear about the severe cognitive impairment. His Wechsler Adult Intelligence Scale – III (Wechsler, 1997a) total IQ score was 58. There were neither significant differences between the four index scores nor the individual subtests. His performance was just, well, flat – similarly to the Wechsler Memory Scale – III (Wechsler, 1997b). All the memory index scores were similar to the Wechsler Adult Intelligence Scale scores. Looking at the results, the testing continued to feel a bit pointless, and time was running out. A test of executive function was needed, just to complete the picture. A Wisconsin Card Sorting Test (Heaton et al., 2003) seemed sensible, and as a computerised test, easy to administer. David failed to understand the task and was clearly baffled by the problem to be solved. Like many patients, he was we by the way things changed, just as he thought he had it figured out. He would probably have done better by simply guessing! Unsurprisingly, on all six domains of the Wisconsin, David's performances were below the fifth percentile.

The next time that David attended an appointment was for feedback on his neuropsychological test results. He arrived on time, was neatly dressed and seemed quite attentive when I told him about his results. Now, like many clinicians, I don't enjoy giving bad news. Accordingly, I tried to be as sensitively as possible, and explained to David that he unfortunately had very severe cognitive impairment. Unsurprisingly, given his apathy and general lack of initiation, he seemed relatively unmoved by this bad news. Or perhaps he also had problems with self-awareness or insight, not an uncommon consequence of traumatic brain injury. I explained to David that I would be seeing him again, after he had seen our neuropsychiatrist. The purpose of our next few appointments, I explained, would be to help him to work around some of his cognitive problems, thereby trying to reduce their impact on his everyday life. These, I suspected, must have been considerable. I felt very sorry for David when he looked at me in silence when I asked him if he had any questions. We arranged that I would see him again on the same day he was coming to hospital for an MRI scan and his appointment with our neuropsychiatrist, in about a fortnight.

The only problem was that, in NHS parlance, David was a DNA (Did not attend). We sent him another appointment. This resulted in another DNA with me, but at least he did manage to see the neuropsychiatrist later that day. Apparently, David missed his train to the hospital, and had to catch a later (afternoon) train. The neuropsychiatrist said that he was not quite sure why David was so severely mentally impaired and slow, because he did not think he was depressed. And he had certainly seen patients with more severe brain injuries who were not as compromised functionally and cognitively. He thought that the MRI would shed light on the issue. But David did not attend his appointment for his MRI brain a month later. Life in the clinic went on, and David got 'lost to follow-up'. Many other patients took his place. And before too long, after about six months, David also got lost to consciousness. New patients and other dilemmas quickly started dominating my, and my colleagues', daily thoughts and our ward rounds.

But then, like a ghost from the past, David returned to our clinic, about a year after I first saw him. Not that he reappeared *in person*, but he certainly re-entered our consciousness. And with a bang!

I first noticed a fat, brown, official-looking envelope, when the neuropsychiatrist asked me to talk about one of my patients. Oh no, what is this about, has someone killed someone. Or done something dreadful which I could, or should, have predicted? He asked me if I could remember someone called David. I must have looked blank, but that was probably just anxiety, interfering with thinking while I was catastrophising about disaster. He reminded me that David was the young man with the diffuse axonal injury, the one I'd tested a few months ago. Instantly relief washed over me. Yes, of course, I remembered him very clearly. He was the one with the very low scores on formal neuropsychological testing. Did I know, the neuropsychiatrist said, that David was involved in a court case?

After my heart rate shot up, and then dropped enough to think straight, I hesitantly asked what the case was about? Most clinicians don't enjoy being dragged into giving evidence in court cases. But David's court case, by the sound of it, was simply to determine the level of damages to award for his brain injury. I almost laughed with relief. Unfortunately, the neuropsychiatrist's expression was not even slightly conducive to smiling. Was I aware that it was a huge claim, for £2 million, and that he (the neuropsychiatrist) had been asked to provide evidence for in court? Also, did I know that David never had his MRI, and that there was only the referrer's 'clinical diagnosis' of diffuse axonal injury? Yes, I did remember all of this. For once I felt useful. Sure, I'd heard everything my neuropsychiatry colleague was saying, and I really did share his apprehension. But I reassured him that we had objective data, *evidence* supporting our diagnosis of a severe traumatic brain injury, and associated significant cognitive impairment. It was now my turn to ask a question. Did he forget that I had performed a full neuropsychological testing?

No, he had not forgotten, and to be completely frank with me, the results were part of his worries, he replied. The other major headache was the absence of any neuroimaging. He did not like going to court, and definitely not when he was not sure of his facts. He reminded me it was *he* who had to go and stand in the dock, and not me. Was I sure of my results? The test scores were very low, and hard to map onto some other facts. For example, did David get to hospital on his own? In fact, how did he manage to live independently at all? I reminded him that David was in fact not living independently, and that he was living with his parents. And that neuropsychological testing was anyway much more sensitive than neuroimaging, and that I had done years, and years of testing by now. He was still not convinced. How did I know David was not like this *before* the injury? And in particular, how did I know he was not exaggerating his difficulties? He wasn't suggesting that David did *not* have a traumatic brain injury, but he was not sure of the magnitude of his impairments.

The conversation with my colleague was becoming ever so slightly annoying. I explained that in clinical neuropsychology we can test for pre-morbid levels of functions, with for example tests of reading ability. These are based on the assumption that language is a 'hold function', meaning it is considered to be relatively more resistant to neurological illness and injury. Did I test for it, he asked? No, because there are other methods, based on demographics, and had he forgotten that David had actually achieved two A levels? Furthermore, David was so slow; it would have been impractical to put him through unnecessary and time-consuming tests. Fair enough, the neuropsychiatrist conceded, but how did I know David gave his best during my tests. This was easy to explain. I told him that there is a whole science around effort testing in clinical neuropsychology. And that it was based upon chance-level performance, coupled with the unlikely occurrence that someone can perform at below chance level on forced choice paradigms.

The neuropsychiatrist looked relieved. He asked if David's results on effort testing showed anything suspicious, or suggestive of possible underperformance. I reminded my colleague that as an experienced clinical neuropsychologist I could decide what to test, and when. David had a documented diffuse axonal injury, and his clinical presentation was compatible with this diagnosis. There was no *need* to test David for effort. That was reserved for say when someone who had suffered a concussion claims to present with a dementia. The neuropsychiatrist looked a little bit stunned. Well, I tried to reassure him, not as dramatic as a concussion presenting as dementia, but obviously effort testing was reserved for when there is a clear external factor (of gain), and the diagnosis and level of reported impairment does not add up. I did the testing my way, based on lots of clinical experience, and he needed not to worry about a thing. David had severe cognitive impairment. He asked me if I was sure. I said I was. From my perspective, everything was clear, and my findings would be helpful for David's case.

The court hearing did in fact bring clarity. But not the sort of clarity I had wished for. Expert evidence was presented by independent practitioners that David most likely did sustain a traumatic brain injury. There indeed was a documented period of loss of consciousness of about two hours, and a subsequent period of confusion and disorientation lasting between one and two days. However, both his CT and MRI scans, requested by the independent clinicians, were reported as normal. An occupational therapy assessment at David's home showed that he was capable of quite a bit more functional independence on activities of daily living than suggested by his reported cognitive difficulties. Formal neuropsychological testing was not repeated. And the clinical neuropsychologist abandoned further testing after David spectacularly failed on the Test of Memory Malingering (Tombaugh, 1996). My colleague, the neuropsychiatrist, told me that it was one of his worst days during his career, appearing in court during David's case for compensation.

3. Error

With the benefit of hindsight, the mistakes made in David's case are glaringly obvious. Failure to get access to any imaging findings is a clear example. Had I seen the (close to) normal scans, I would have thought twice about how they failed to map to the clinical presentation. And the test presentation, so uniformly terrible, in someone who appeared to live with a degree of independence? Or, indeed, someone who may well have come to the hospital, on time, apparently unaided? Why hadn't I asked the questions? There are also other errors of clinical reasoning. For example, David had no loss of sense of smell or taste, in the context of a supposed severe traumatic brain injury? Despite that I knew about the olfactory bulb and tracts, and the sphenoid ridges in TBI. . . . This should have been a patient where there was some ambiguity about a diagnosis, or the severity of its symptoms, in which case I might have well tested for effort. Indeed, the British Psychological Society (2009) advises that, while there are exclusions to the general rule, effort testing should *routinely* be administered during formal neuropsychological assessment.

What then contributed to my blindness? One cannot rule out the issue of time here. Testing him was exhausting, and I had other, apparently more pressing cases. And then there was over reliance on an *assumed* diagnosis, without checking all the objective evidence for it having been made. Too much was also made of experience, and an overconfidence in deciding when, and when not, effort testing would be necessary. Another obvious mistake was the failure to think more clearly about David's premorbid level of functioning. I accepted far too casually David's word for having passed two A levels, without checking for example the school records or reports. That he completed secondary school, despite one of the lowest IQ level that I'd ever scored? Meaning, of course, that it would have been sensible to administer a test of premorbid function?

There was also a broader, almost more philosophical factor which contributed to my blatant errors of clinical reasoning. It is not helpful to be too closely aligned as a clinical neuropsychologist to being a member of the 'School of rehabilitation' or the 'College of assessment'. Some posts may well require more of one or the other aspects of professional practice, the effective clinical neuropsychologist should always remain up to date in *both*. My identity in this case was, alas, too clearly as a 'rehabilitationist', and I would have done well to focus more on the importance of assessment. To my eternal regret, I did it 'my way', rather than the correct way.

4. Reflection

Neuropsychological assessment is one of the activities that define clinical neuropsychology as a profession with a unique identity. No other allied health professions, nor medical colleagues such as neurologists and neuropsychiatrists, perform cognitive testing to the level of sophistication that is so specific. Neuropsychological assessment is also integral to the process of rehabilitation, by means of its ability to more accurately identify patients' cognitive strengths and weaknesses. But psychological tests can be complex to interpret. Test performance on the individual cognitive domains should always be interpreted in the broader contexts of patients' own baseline, general ability, as well as crucially, their effort.

Reflecting on the mistakes made at several time points in the case of David, the clinician would have done much better to philosophically and professionally embrace testing as integral to the role of the clinical neuropsychologist, even though the personal identity of the clinician in this example was as a 'rehabilitationist', rather than a diagnostician. The main learning point? Never perform an assessment 'my way', when research, evidence-base and expert consensus can so much better inform our practice.

References

British Psychological Society (2009). *Assessment of Effort in Clinical Testing of Cognitive Functioning for Adults*. Leicester: British Psychological Society.

Heaton, R. R. & PAR Staff (2003). *WCST: CV4 Wisconsin Card Sorting Test: Computer Version 4*. Lutz, FL: Psychological Assessment Resources.

Tombaugh, T. N. (1996). *Test of Memory Malingering*. North Tonawanda, NY: Multi-Health Systems.

Walsh, K. (1992). Some gnomes worth knowing. *Clinical Neuropsychologist*, *6*(2), 119–133. https://doi.org/10.1080/13854049208401849

Wechsler, D. (1997a). *Wechsler Adult Intelligence Scale III*. San Antonio, TX: Psychological Corporation.

Wechsler, D. (1997b). *Wechsler Memory Scale III*. San Antonio, TX: Psychological Corporation.

9 Rudderless rehabilitation

Rudi Coetzer

'We learn from failure, not from success'.

—Bram Stoker, Lady Athlyne

1. Situation

Another day, there was another referral letter. Requests to 'make things better' arrive one after the other in the average clinical neuropsychologist's in tray. Especially for those of us working in more rehabilitation oriented clinical services. Often these referrals come from within the multidisciplinary team, rather than necessarily always an external source. Therein often is contained the 'subtext' for the referral. It is not uncommon for patients referred for neuropsychological treatment to have a complex combination of social, psychological, and physical problems, and as a result to have become 'stuck' in their rehabilitation within the multidisciplinary team. In other words, quite frequently there is a rather desperate undertone to the referrers' requests, bordering on a plea, to help, anything, just to 'make things a bit better'. It is exactly these emotive pleas which can at times make us forget some of the underpinning knowledge we learned all those years ago while still in training.

Early in our careers, between the cyclical (and normal) crises of confidence and self-doubt, the average neuropsychologist tends to have a very strong desire, bordering on pathological anxiety and guilt, to make a worthwhile contribution to the work of the teams where they are employed. Where might this originate from? By far the most difficult part of clinical training is selection, with all sorts of challenges to secure a training place against the overwhelming odds of competing against literally hundreds of other extremely well-qualified applicants. While the three years[1] of non-stop daily stress of lectures, exams and seeing patients is hard, it is not even nearly as challenging as going through selection in the first instance. Perhaps after selection, it is this sense of disbelief that leaves us with a desire to demonstrate that during training, and after qualifying, that we are valuable, that we *deserve* to be clinicians. And that we are therefore able to further the collective aims of the team, that we are effective with caring for patients, so that . . . if we are completely honest, we can earn the very precious currency called *credibility*. It is a rite of passage, to earn

DOI:10.4324/9781003300748-9

your 'wings', and become part of the clan. Recently clinically qualified, we have high levels of academic knowledge, and mountains of enthusiasm, but low experience of clinical work. Unfortunately, the missing crucial ingredient here is experience. But good we must do. Is this then the career stage where the newly appointed, inexperienced clinical neuropsychologist is often loved by the team for their hard work, and enthusiasm to 'always say yes', but equally also seen as perhaps slightly naive? It is of course an essential professional developmental stage, to gradually balance naivety with a little bit of realism.

2. Example

Mair was 47 when she suffered a right middle cerebral artery stroke. At the time of her stroke, Mair was employed part-time as an accountant's assistant. It was a small firm dealing mainly with tax returns, and they were based not too far from where Mair lived. She had been working for them 12 years. Mair was at work when she started feeling unwell, with an excruciating headache. Mair said it was a 'headache like never before', and that she could not properly move her left arm and leg. At some point, she thought that she felt so ill that she vomited, which was when one of the accountants realised that something was desperately wrong. But from here on things are a bit hazy for Mair, and she couldn't quite recall everything. In fact, an ambulance was called, and Mair was taken directly to hospital. After triage, and an initial clinical examination in A & E, a CT scan of the brain confirmed that she had suffered a stroke. Mair was admitted to hospital, initially to a medical ward, but after two days was transferred to the hospital's on-site rehabilitation team.

After spending four weeks in the hospital's inpatient stroke rehabilitation unit, the clinical team felt that Mair had probably made enough progress with her physical rehabilitation to go home. At this point, she was independent for all activities of daily living, although she did have a mild residual left sided weakness, some memory problems, and 'low mood'. In any case, that is what the referral to our community-based brain injury rehabilitation service suggested. The referral was accepted, and Mair was offered an initial screening. Based on this clinical assessment, Mair was offered further physiotherapy, occupational therapy, and an appointment with our psychiatrist, in view of her suspected presentation with depression post-stroke. Shortly after these commenced, she was also seen by the social worker for a first assessment of any financial or other difficulties. Although Mair was seen very soon post-discharge, and had a good few appointments, things were not quite going according to plan. But at least it was still (relatively) early days, at least as things go in post-acute rehab.

However, the team thought that Mair was not engaging that well with her post-acute rehab, and failing to make the gains anticipated. At a weekly clinical team meeting a couple of months after she was referred to us, the occupational therapist and physiotherapist asked if I would be willing to see her. They explained that from their perspective, Mair seemed 'stuck' for some reason. The occupational therapist thought, for example, that she was not willing to work towards a phased return to employment. Something was blocking her progress in this area. In her view, Mair was depressed, and often became tearful during their rehabilitation sessions. The physiotherapist had an altogether different take on the formulation. In her view Mair had poor initiation or motivation, and memory difficulties, with both contributing to her failure to systematically engage with her physiotherapy. To further evidence her point, the physiotherapist said that she had also spoken to the psychiatrist, who thought that Mair was *not* depressed. The psychiatrist posited that, instead of a mood disorder, Mair might have pre-existing personality traits of being more dependent. She (the psychiatrist) also did wonder about Mair's 'insight'. Well, of course a psychiatrist would say that. While the physiotherapist and occupational therapist did not agree as regards a formulation of Mair's presentation, one thing they did agree on. She needed to see the clinical neuropsychologist, sooner, rather than later.

The first appointment did not start brilliantly. Mair almost immediately started crying when I asked what her main difficulties were, and how I might help her. Fortunately, the consultation room had a box of tissues readily to hand. If only achieving good psychological outcomes were as simple as drying patients' tears. . . . Mair told me between tearful episodes, that she was very worried. I asked what was playing on her mind? She replied that she may be evicted from her home, unless the social worker urgently filled in her forms for her. Returning to work would then be the obvious solution? However, when I asked Mair about her plans about returning to work, she said that she couldn't recall seeing the occupational therapist. After prompting, she did seem to remember meeting someone, perhaps a therapist of sorts, but appeared to be confused as to who did what? It was difficult to know who was who, she said, because nobody really wore distinctive uniforms. Anyway, she did not find the interventions and support particularly helpful. Her arm and leg were uncomfortable, with constant pins and needles. How could she do the exercises or try to go back to work? What about the psychiatrist, I asked, might that be helpful? Mair looked at me in surprise. She has not seen the psychiatrist before today – she thought that *I* was the psychiatrist. Ah, it all suddenly made sense to me. Mair has significant problems with new learning and retention, which fits in with her stroke and explains why she was 'not engaging'.

The occupational therapist and physiotherapist were impressed by my diagnostic acumen. It took me only one session to determine that poor memory explained her lack of engagement. I had a plan. Memory rehab will be the first step on the path to Mair's re-engagement with her rehabilitation. At our next appointment, Mair did not cry at all. In fact, she did not express *any* strong emotions. She said she was hoping to go back to work before too long. Did she remember our previous session? And that we were going to look at some strategies to help her with her memory? She didn't resist the plan, and we duly started discussing some strategies she might find helpful. Like many people, Mair was already using her smartphone, for not only communication and social media, but also using its calendar function. This was then a good starting point: a compensatory approach, and ecologically valid one, to managing the memory difficulties. As my physiotherapy colleague had pointed out a couple of weeks ago. Mair managed to quickly figure out how she could better use her phone's calendar function, and link this up with additional reminders via text messaging. We also discussed the possible value of keeping a small pocket diary, perhaps as a backup. Or maybe even as a more narrative-based tool to help with developing an ongoing sense of continuity, and with progress made in rehabilitation. Something she could refer back to. Plus, a diary doesn't have a battery that can run flat, I added. Things were looking up.

The crash came much sooner than anticipated. Less than a week after our previous meeting, Mair phoned to ask if she could see me a bit earlier, as she was 'worrying herself to death'. Well, that made perfect sense. Memory problems are associated with anxiety. Plus, Mair, now being able to compensate for her poor retention, would of course have *access* to stuff to worry about. She arrived for her appointment on time. It was noticeable that her walking and general mobility was still rapidly improving. It was now difficult to see any obvious signs of her initial left-sided weakness. In fact, the more noticeable observation was now about her anxiety, rather than low mood or poor mobility. I thought things were going well, that she was using the memory strategies we covered. Was she looking forward to trying to get to work? Yes, that is all true, Mair agreed, but she was feeling very lonely. Really lonely. Nobody's been to visit. Even her partner has not been to see her as regularly, and she found it very difficult to make decisions without her input. Ah, how could I have missed that! Social isolation after stroke, or any type of acquired brain injury, is a well-known nettle out there in the world where our patients live. Thus, Mair would be an ideal candidate for some of our post-acute rehabilitation groups, which have a strong focus on social cohesion. In particular, the woodwork group offered weekly occupational therapy input, and loads of opportunity for social interaction. And as a bonus, Mair seemed really keen to go.

Only problem was Mair did not actually attend the woodwork groups. We discussed the reasons for this happening. The more Mair spoke, the more convinced I became that this was obviously as a result of her loss of confidence. Reflecting on my previous discussions with the team, in particular the occupational therapist, I could now appreciate how loss of confidence could easily be mistaken for depression. And to be honest, loss of confidence was not infrequently itself a *feature* of depression. Nevertheless, I was still convinced Mair was not depressed. It is not rocket science – if we have memory problems, we become anxious, and . . . lose our confidence. I tried to reassure Mair that I had a plan. We will work together for a few sessions to help her become a bit more confident. When she asked how this will work, I explained that sometimes it helps to talk to someone neutral about what worries us, and specifically also about the thoughts which make us a bit more nervous, low, or result in us avoiding doing certain things. I even gave it the fancy sounding name: Cognitive Behavioural Therapy, or 'CBT' for short. Mair appeared to be really impressed, and keen to engage in therapy. I was very pleased that her sense of hope had returned. That in itself was a good sign that her confidence had the potential to improve.

Mair grasped the rationale of CBT without too much difficulty. We spent the next four sessions making sure that she had good mastery of the main techniques of CBT. I gradually started to increase the emphasis on behavioural activation, including behavioural experiments. After a couple of easy low-risk homework assignments, for example to re-engage socially with her neighbour by inviting her over for coffee, I thought Mair was ready for 'the big two'. She would go to the woodwork group, and commence a more concerted phased return to work. It did not go well. Mair went to the woodwork group and had little problems with the simple tasks. However, she spectacularly failed whenever 'multi-tasking' and complex processing was required. She could remember the separate steps involved in making a chess board but could not integrate everything. And it was a disaster when she was distracted. The problem also very glaringly revealed itself in social situations. Mair just could not keep track of group conversations. She got lost in who said what, she 'fell behind' while 'trying to figure things out', and then 'just shut up'. All of this I learnt about through feedback from the occupational therapists based at the woodwork workshop. Mair had ceased to attend. They were also very concerned that she 'did not quite grasp' the nature of her problems, saying she was 'fine', and that she 'just had a lot on her mind' at the moment. Will I please see what I can do about it when I saw her for her next appointment . . . ?

Mair's next appointment was our most important. She burst out in tears when I gently tried to enquire how things had been for her, and how she was finding the woodwork group. She just sobbed. Between her tears, she said that things had never been easy for her. She relied on her partner, and work to help her with complicated stuff, and then this stroke. Why did it happen? Thought she'd be better by now? In fact, she had been feeling fine for quite some time now, her walking and use of her left hand have been fine. She also noted that she'd seen many patients who were much worse than her, with quite obvious physical difficulties. In fact, the woodwork was very busy, lots of people all talking at the same time. Suddenly Mair stopped sobbing. She looked at me, almost as if slightly surprised. It was at that moment that she asked *the question*. Quite obviously perplexed, she asked me what was *wrong*, why was she struggling so much? It was now six months since her stroke. At the hospital, they said by six months or so things should be fine. And yet . . . she was still not back at work. The woodwork groups did not quite work out, and she did not enjoy being there with the other people. She wondered what was going on. Nothing was going to plan. Suddenly she looked really frightened. Was there something *wrong* with her?

3. Error

Mair's question cuts to the heart of what has gone wrong here. Her rehab has been driven by everything, except . . . a sound theoretical or clinical model of neuropsychological intervention. Yes, of course there is something *wrong* with her. She suffered a stroke, and broadly speaking has impairments and associated disabilities deemed reasonably compatible with her lesion. But any good neuropsychological intervention should start with a good assessment of the patient's presentation, history and impairments. The latter would include changes in behaviour, emotion and cognition. Rather than *guess* these as the consultations go along, Mair should have been assessed more systematically, including a thorough bedside cognitive assessment, or even better, a formal neuropsychological assessment. Without this, we simply don't know the cognitive impairments of our patients, their strengths, and quite often, what might *really* sit behind their anxiety or depression for example. That was the first error in Mair's care: a lack of assessment and testing to identify *what* exactly was 'wrong', and what needed to be targeted during her neuropsychological rehabilitation.

Something else that was very wrong in this case description was the absence of any theoretical model of rehabilitation to guide the formulation, interventions, and feedback to the team (MacNiven, 2016). We cannot rehabilitate what we don't understand, and we need models of the processes and problems we are targeting during our interventions. Theoretical models should be the compass of the clinical neuropsychologist. They incorporate concepts such as spontaneous recovery versus restorative and compensatory approaches to reduce impairments, or the consequences of impairments – disability. Sometimes a restitution (restorative) approach might well be indicated. Notably, Donald Hebb's work during the late 1940s continues to influence some aspects of rehabilitation to this day. However, it is often a compensatory and adjustment approach which is required. And we also know that some impairments can be better addressed with some approaches and not others. The elephant in the room of this case was impulsive, haphazard and frequent changes in formulation between sessions with Mair. That was hopefully plainly obvious to most readers. But yet again something feels wrong here, almost as if a key ingredient is missing? As they say, in theory models and systems work very well, but once they leave the safe confines of the written page, some though (not all) can flounder.

And finally, Mair, through her question, shows us the most important aspect of this error. Most neuropsychological rehabilitation models now at least take into consideration, or often place centrally, the issue of patient self-awareness, often previously described as 'insight'. In Mair's case the interventions offered to her were all too often reactive, with little consideration of her understanding of her weaknesses and strengths. Even worse than that, Mair was never formally assessed by a neuropsychologist. Worryingly, it was not actually *known* what her real cognitive and other impairments were, at least objectively. A structured assessment of mood and anxiety was also not conducted. What if Mair *said* that her memory was fine? Was her memory (and which part of memory . . .) really as good as before the stroke. Alternatively, did she have problems of self-awareness, so that her subjective account was inaccurate? Actually, who knows?

The problem with self-awareness is that not only it is there, everywhere, in the consultation room but also *invisible*. The only remedy is to assess the patient, and ideally relatives, friends or carers, who knows them well, and knew them *before* the neurological problems.

On the topic of challenges, self-awareness is often not static. After an acquired brain injury, it tends to evolve. It may be very difficult to engage patients in their rehabilitation during the early stages, when they may not think there is anything wrong with them. However, as they start to fail, and experience repeated environmental feedback, self-awareness can change. No wonder that Mair eventually asked whether there was something wrong with her.

4. Reflection

'Rudderless rehabilitation' is one of that easily fallen into traps for the new, and even for the experienced, clinical neuropsychologist. At times, our desire to show that we are worthy of having been selected to become clinicians, to do good, to help others, blinds us to the basic models that normally should underpin our interventions. In other situations, we feel a desperate need to 'prove' to our non-neuropsychology colleagues that our input to the team is valuable. These, and other, factors sometimes make us vulnerable to go *off-piste* when planning (or not) our interventions. At times, in desperation, we may use a shotgun approach – to fire everything at the problem, and see what hits the target.

There are many things I could have done better in this case description. With the benefit of hindsight, it was fatal not to perform a neuropsychological assessment, to guide Mair's rehabilitation. The feedback of her results directly to Mair could also have told me a lot more than merely what her strengths and weaknesses were. It would have provided an early opportunity to gauge her understanding of her difficulties, or even possibly her denial of them. I absolutely should have asked her what her rehabilitation goals were. Even though I should have known better, there was also a lack of top-down thinking in this case. What could one rightly expect after a right middle cerebral artery stroke? This would have complemented testing, by providing more specific hypotheses to test. Who knows what might have happened? One thing is almost certain though, her path of rehab would have taken a different direction.

In addition, I could have communicated better with the clinical team. Besides the two short conversations with the physiotherapist and occupational therapist, I never really found out first hand from the rest of the team what *they* thought. In particular, I had never asked the psychiatrist what their views were. I feel guilty about all of these mistakes. One of the fundamental requirements of multi-disciplinary teams is to work to the same goals for a given patient. It is here where theoretical models and combined formulations are very important. Every member of the team understands the overarching reasons for doing things in a certain way, and why. This is crucial in neuropsychological reha-bilitation models – especially where self-awareness and psychotherapy is central to how we structure interventions (see Prigatano, 1989, 1999, for more of this linked to holistic rehabilitation). I now wish that I had checked in more frequently with the clinical team, and listened to what they thought.

A final improvement in the management of the case would have been to invite Mair's partner or other close person, in for an interview (with Mair's consent, of course), to determine what *really* was different from before, and what was actually happening at home. This information would have helped me to form an even better picture of Mair's difficulties, how she viewed then, what maintained them and what were potential protective factors.

One of the first steps in patients' rehabilitation is come to some agreement of what they, and we, see as their difficulties, what (if any) needs there are for intervention, and their motivation to engage with rehabilitation. Yes, to some degree this is determined by testing and assessment. But ultimately these findings need to be translated to the worlds of our patients, where they live, what they do and who they socially interact with. This helps to make the rehabilitation goals ecologically valid, for both parties. Without this mutually agreed, negotiated, starting point (sometimes referred to as 'contracting') in rehabilitation, both parties are at risk of remaining in the dark as to what they are doing in the consultation room. Alas, therefore, 'Rehabilitation in the dark' risks producing little beyond what can be accounted for by spontaneous recovery. Our patients deserve better. And we, as clinicians, will then have earned the ability to be part of a team that is making a difference.

Note

1 We refer here to the standard UK model of training, which is a 3-year Doctorate (D.Clin.Psy), consisting of a mixture of lectures, essays, examinations, clinical placements and research projects.

References

MacNiven, J. A. B. (Ed.) (2016). *Neuropsychological formulation. A clinical casebook*. New York: Springer.

Prigatano, G. P. (1989). Work, love, and play after brain injury. *Bulletin of the Menninger Clinic*, 53 (5): 414–431.

Prigatano, G. P. (1999). *Principles of neuropsychological rehabilitation*. New York: Oxford University Press.

10 Thinking inside the box

Oliver Turnbull, Leanne Rowlands **&** *Rudi Coetzer*

'The world is like a game of chess, varying at every move'.

—William Scarborough (1875)

1. Situation

'Resources are finite'. Does this ring a bell? Clinical neuropsychologists hate hearing this assertion from our funders, or senior management, irrespective of whether we are working in publicly funded or independent healthcare settings. Nevertheless, many clinical neuropsychologists would secretly admit that this common management phrase is, unfortunately, simply a statement of fact – a reflection of reality, nothing more, nothing less. While we might protest, deep down we do realise that often *more* has to be delivered to our patients, but with fewer resources – within reason, of course. We also understand that asking for yet more staff, to provide more input, is not always the best or even most creative solution to service development (see, e.g. Coetzer, 2014; Coetzer et al., 2003). Service development and improvement entails more than securing ever increasing amounts of money, as some of us have learnt the hard way. The sobering truth is that, more often than most would admit, not all the money in the world, nor all the staff that can be recruited, can 'make better' many of the neurological illnesses and injuries we see every day. Instead, service development is often about doing things differently, but better for our patients.

Developing efficient clinical services entails putting together several pieces of a very complex puzzle. To make things even more complex, it is also unfortunately not a static puzzle. Many factors, for example changes in best practice over time, new therapies or altered needs of patients, make sure the puzzle is always a moving target. While a basic level of resource allocation is always the minimum starting point, it is what comes *after* this which is often really challenging. At this stage of service development and improvement, helpful strategies may include working differently, and smarter, with what is available. Some of the approaches to thinking about improving efficiency also include a consideration of the 'dose' effect, or working out the ideal frequency and length of time of therapeutic input. Too little, and the effect or outcome is not good enough. Too much, and the outcome, while perhaps better, costs too much.

DOI:10.4324/9781003300748-10

Sometimes it is also very helpful to try and find new partners (e.g. outside of the hospital system) to collaborate with. Another consideration is economies of scale. One of the most commonly employed strategies is, of course, the use of groups to deliver rehabilitation therapies. The maths is simple – one therapist, simultaneously seeing several patients, versus a ratio of one-to-one. This chapter describes our journey, and some lessons.

2. Example

Ours was going to be the mother of all psycho-education group interventions. Evidence-based, research informed, creatively designed and delivered. We were aware that most community brain injury services were providing psycho-education groups. But we had discovered, through an initial literature review, that few appeared to have ever looked more closely into the rationale, or the evidence base, for providing these groups.

Thus, while group therapy is widely used in brain injury rehabilitation services, research has lagged behind on its actual effectiveness (Hammond et al., 2015; Tuckman, 1965). Many services also appear to have a 'homegrown' approach to running group programmes, which are developed in line with expert experiences and opinions, but are seldom evaluated empirically (see Patterson et al., 2016, for a review). Perhaps because psycho-education makes a lot of intuitive clinical sense, it has always been *assumed* to be a robust tool for helping patients with brain injury. Assumed to be able to help them better manage some of their difficulties, including memory problems, or poor social skills – hence the popularity of psycho-education groups with clinicians. But we live in a world of evidence-based medicine, and we would do well to try to back up our intuitions.

There was clearly a niche in the market, and we were well placed to capitalise. Could this also be a way to improve the effectiveness of group therapy provision, while *reducing* the cost of service-delivery? So, our clinical service lead (RC) successfully teamed up with its long-standing local University partner (OT), and together secured some funding to look at further developing and improving the delivery of psycho-education groups (carried out by LR).

Our service has something of a reputation for especially focusing on patients attending post-acute rehabilitation at the hospital (Coetzer et al., 2018). This principle, to 'Build long-term', has been part of our approach for decades. This seems important, because the provision of support for people with ABI in the *chronic* phase has, alas, been an area of limited emphasis in the literature (Turner-Stokes et al., 2015). Notably, however, many patients' difficulties persist into the chronic phase (Ponsford et al., 2014), and can of course last a life-time.

A second principle that lay behind our approach to psycho-education was a desire to 'Focus on feelings'. The majority of evaluated interventions from the literature have focused on *cognitive* impairment (Bayley et al., 2014; Patterson et al., 2016 for review). Indeed, cognition has traditionally taken precedence in rehabilitation services (Ben-Yishay & Prigatano, 1990; Rohling et al., 2009; Wilson, 1997). More recently, however, there has been an 'emotional turn' in neuropsychological rehabilitation, where greater emphasis is placed on socio-emotional adjustment, and feelings are increasingly at the heart of case formulation (Bowen et al., 2010; Coetzer et al., 2018; Wilson & Betteridge, 2019; Wilson & Gracey, 2009; McDonald, 2017).

Importantly, it is well documented that survivors can experience a range of emotional disorders, most commonly anxiety and depression (Fleminger, 2008; Kreutzer et al., 2001; Rao & Lyketsos, 2000; Scholten et al., 2016). Typically, these emotional difficulties are indeed persistent in the long term (Fleminger, 2008), and represent a substantial unmet need for survivors (Chen et al., 2019; McKevitt et al., 2011; Walsh et al., 2015). To counter this, there is a developing line of evidence on the role of *positive* experiences (e.g. support of family and friends; Fraas & Calvert, 2009; meaningful activities; Downing et al., 2021; Lyon et al., 2021) and psychological approaches (e.g. optimism, problem-focused coping; Glintborg & Hansen, 2016; Shotton et al., 2007), in promoting recovery and adjustment. Related to this, emotion regulation after ABI has received limited attention in the literature, though the last decade has seen some progress here, including work from our group, (Bechara, 2004; Beer & Lombardo, 2007; Salas, 2012; Salas et al., 2014, 2019).

On the question of practicalities, our clinical service was already well versed in delivering psycho-education groups to our head-injured patients. So, for once here in the hospital, enthusiasm and optimism were not in short supply. We knew how to run psycho-education, and our new plan would, we hoped, improve what we were providing to our patients.

This then was our goal: a novel approach to rehabilitation, focusing on feelings, with a positive psychology emphasis, using the well-established group psycho-education approach. And we needed to make sure to evaluate the study, and publish it! This wouldn't be a cost-saving exercise, but instead an opportunity to do things in a much better way.

3. Unexpected outcomes

The project is now completed, and the work is in various stages of publication (Rowlands et al., 2019, 2020, 2021). This chapter does not focus on any 'mistakes' from the work. But it does describe three outcomes of the study which were genuinely surprising to us. Despite many decades of experience in neuropsychology, these outcomes were each unexpected, and made us re-think some key principles that underlie rehabilitation.

Groups are themselves therapeutic agents

There is half a century worth of research on what makes psychotherapy effective (e.g. Roth & Fonagy, 2006). Most of this has been on individual, one-to-one work, and heavily biased towards psychotherapy with 'psychiatric', rather than neurological, populations. Here, it seems clear that the most important variable predicting progress is the phenomenon sometimes described as the therapeutic alliance – the extent to which the patient feels that they are working together with the therapist in addressing the patient's problems (Martin et al., 2000). What is less clear is the extent to which this principle applies to *group* processes. No doubt having a helpful facilitator can make all the difference to the work of the group? But what is role of the group itself?

The results of the study were a genuine surprise to us. The extent to which the group was perceived to have worked together (group cohesion) was an important predictor of patient outcome, and clearly statistically significant (Rowlands et al., in preparation). On the other hand, patient evaluation of the therapeutic alliance was that it was a far *less* important predictor, and was even negatively associated with some outcomes. This feeling was summed up in some of the qualitative data produced by the patients. 'We're all in the same boat', said one patient. It was only someone else who had a brain injury, they felt, who could properly understand their situation, and empathise with them in a way that was helpful. Socialising with similar others helped generate a sense of normality in the group, where patients felt free and comfortable to be themselves. Though we were less aware of this work, this effect has been found for other group interventions, so that groups help survivors to adjust to a 'new normal', assist with the complex process of identity reconstruction (Couchman et al., 2014; Lexell et al., 2013), and can help avoid social isolation after ABI (Salas et al., 2018).

Anticipation is a great friend of happiness

We were always interested for our programme to frame the emotional world of our patients in a more positive light. Taking our lead from the ideas behind positive psychology (Seligman, 2011), and not over-focus on difficulties, but instead emphasise the positive. So we decided to introduce the well-known '*Three good things*' approach (Seligman et al., 2005) to our rehabilitation programme. Three good things invites people to write down three positive experiences that they have had during the day, thinking about them, in a brief period of reflection, towards the end of the day.

You might wonder, of course, about why spending just a few of minutes in the evening might improve overall happiness? It may well be because, when done regularly and well, *Three good things* doesn't just simply last for a few minutes before bedtime. Importantly, it means that the patient is spending lots of the day *looking out* for things which may later make it to their bedtime list. 'That was a fun conversation, perhaps I can use that on my list?' 'That tree looks amazing, perhaps I'll use that later?' And so on. The approach is effective in large part because it encourages the focus of attention towards positive experiences throughout the day, rather than patients ruminating on the problems and challenges in their lives.

It may well also be helpful because it favours an approach towards anticipation. This is increasingly well understood as being mediated by the brain's premier positive emotion system, sometimes described as wanting (Berridge, 2009), or SEEKING (Panksepp, 2004). This (dopamine mediated) system is clearly activated by all forms of exploration in the world, and the anticipation that comes with new objects and experiences (Schultz et al., 1997). Clearly, if patients are looking out for things during the day which they can use in the evening, then this seems likely to be recruiting our anticipatory seeking system. For these reasons we were hopeful that *Three good things* would be a useful part of our therapeutic programme, and that patients would save up their good experiences for their evenings.

We were genuinely surprised at the way that these good experiences panned out in our group setting. The surprise was not that the patients recorded the positive experiences at the end of the day. But something *additional* seemed to happen in relation to the group. Not only were they recording their experiences for *themselves*, but they were then holding on to them, and bringing these positive experiences into their weekly group meetings. This is something that we don't think has been tried, or at least reported, in the literature.

There are, of course, many important implications for this form of sharing. It means that our patients are holding on their positive experiences for much longer. Not just for a few hours until bedtime, but for a few days until the next group meeting. Notably, and perhaps more importantly, they are also bringing these positive experiences not just to themselves but to the wider group. This serves as a reminder of the way that groups can go awry. All trainees will have sat in group therapy sessions in which patients have produced a long list of complaints about the challenges of their lives. These are undoubtedly valid feelings, but they can tend to lower the tone, and simply remind the group of the difficulties they face. Imagine, instead, if the group conversation was more upbeat? For us, *Three good things* changed the tenor of the group sessions entirely. Instead of complaints, meetings often became a celebration of the positive things that had happened to members of the group throughout the week – a quite unexpected, and a very positive, outcome.

Simple is good. Simpler is better

The literature on memory rehabilitation after brain injury has had many interesting ideas over the years. It didn't take the field long, for example, to discover that 'practising' memory didn't seem to be very beneficial for patients. It's too much effort, and memory doesn't seem to be a muscle in that way. Instead, the greater gain seems to come from *external* memory aids, an approach that Luria would have been delighted with. In the earlier years, this meant the use of diaries, and other reminders, such as lists and post-it notes. More recently, there has been increasing use of technology, most notably in the form of smartphones. However, both approaches have their downsides, not least, and rather ironically, because patients with memory problems have a worrying habit of forgetting where they *left* their diaries and smartphones.

Our patients were already using these approaches. So we sought to add value by adding an even simpler, and very practical, tool, by suggesting the use of a box. Patients with memory difficulties would be encouraged to find a box, and put it near the front door of their house or flat. Even *in front* of (i.e. on the *inside* of) the door, if need be. These boxes are easy to find, we would say, because those delivery companies give you one *free*, every time they bring you a parcel!

So, when the patient enters their house, they are to be advised to always leave all the important things, like keys, wallet and spectacles, in the box. We emphasised the concepts '*always* leave', and 'leave *all* the things', because habit is really important. This way they always knew where to find objects before they leave home. And if there was something that they needed to, for example, take with them *tomorrow*, then they didn't need to write it down, or log a reminder in their smart phone. Instead, they would go, immediately, and put the 'to be remembered' item in the box. This allowed the box to serving as a sort of memory buffer, holding material that the patient no longer needed to worry about. And the box was a well-*located* memory buffer too, because it served as a practical reminder, as they walked past it, or even *into* it, whenever they were leaving the property. If you can't open the door without looking at the box, or if you have to move it out of the way before opening the door, then forgetfulness is much less likely. A compensatory strategy that's impossible to miss.

This approach was consistent what other things we've tried in rehabilitation, notably trying to find concrete solutions for our patients. Chapter 11 deals with this issue in more detail. So, we were hopeful that our simple approach would turn out to be a useful adjunct to smartphones and diaries.

Once the programme had been implemented, our little box strategy really did exceed our expectations. During the trial, patients regularly reported using the box, and always in a positive light ('it's a game changer', one patient reported). But the real surprise for us came during long-term follow-up, several months or even years later. Speaking to one of us as their clinician (RC), and entirely unprompted, patients regularly reported the box as one of *the* most important things that they had gained from the treatment programme. 'It's been so amazing. I don't know why people didn't tell me about this before?' It was a common refrain. And all from a tool that is effectively free.

4. Reflection

We work so hard to make things better for our patients – often with fairly limited resources at our disposal. Despite this we go on, and try to work even harder. The problem clearly is not as a result of a lack of commitment to our patients and their well-being. But perhaps in the frantic work schedule, we don't pause often enough to reflect on our work – more specifically, to reflect on 'what works for whom?'

Our three 'errors', or unexpected outcomes, speak to the question of why many well-intended rehabilitation interventions often have less than ideal outcomes. First, we feel that some interventions get the 'simplicity-complexity' balance wrong. Too simplistic as regards underpinning theory and research evidence, but too *complex* as regards the actual practical intervention. It produces a lack of generalisation of the rehabilitation gains, and an inability to transfer the new behaviour outside the learning environment (Baer et al., 1968). This can undermine all of our substantial effort, and can undermine the efficacy of our therapeutic work (Newby et al., 2013). We need to ensure that the gains *transfer* to the real world, out there where our patients live. And, importantly, the gains are *sustained*. Too much complexity, and the therapeutic gains made during sessions don't 'travel' very far beyond the clinic. The humble cardboard box is an excellent example of this, and we would do well to think of interventions through the lens of sustainable transfer. What are we doing to ensure that this therapeutic tool will be interesting, practical, simple and perhaps even fun? What will help it 'stick'?

The other unexpected outcome relates, of course, to groups. There is sometimes a perception that group therapy is a way of achieving treatment 'on the cheap'. It generates an impression that a hard-pressed service can only *afford* to deliver group interventions, and that we would work one-to-one if we had more resources. Our data, and the growing literature, suggest that well-managed groups can be a powerful agent in the delivery of therapeutic change.

One important element of this is that these groups can continue to support each other, long after the therapeutic intervention itself is over. We specifically designed our intervention, for example, so that patients shared their contact details (Facebook, WhatsApp, etc.) during the first session. We also focused on the final session, which was themed as a celebration, with food and drink, and the presentation of the certificate. To make it a small graduation ceremony – and in reality these turned out to be lovely events. Importantly, the patients had to work *together* across all the sessions to organise the activities for that final week. This was our attempt to try and build a small community of people who were 'all in the same boat'. A community who would continue to support each other even when the sessions had finished, and would allow the service to build long term.

So, we have moved from a position of accepting groups as standard clinical practice, to becoming genuine enthusiasts for the benefits that groups offer. Indeed, we suspect that, even if we did have more of those 'additional resources' that services dream of, that we would still deliver our psycho-education sessions in groups.

References

Baer, D. M., Wolf, M. M., & Risley, T. R. (1968). Some current dimensions of applied behavior analysis. *Journal of Applied Behavior Analysis, 1*(1), 91.

Bayley, M. T., Tate, R., Douglas, J. M., Turkstra, L. S., Ponsford, J., Stergiou-Kita, M., . . . Bragge, P. (2014). INCOG guidelines for cognitive rehabilitation following traumatic brain injury: Methods and overview. *The Journal of Head Trauma Rehabilitation, 29*(4), 290–306.

Bechara, A. (2004). Disturbances of emotion regulation after focal brain lesions. *International Review of Neurobiology, 62*, 159–193.

Beer, J. S., & Lombardo, M. V. (2007). Insights into emotion regulation from neuropsychology. In J. J. Gross (Ed.), *Handbook of emotion regulation* (pp. 69–86). New York: The Guilford Press.

Ben-Yishay, Y., & Prigatano, G. P. (1990). Cognitive remediation. In M. Rosenthal, M. R. Bond, E. R. Griffith, & J. D. Miller (Eds.), *Rehabilitation of the adult and child with traumatic brain injury* (pp. 393–409). Philadelphia, PA: F. A. Davis.

Berridge, K. C. (2009). Wanting and liking: Observations from the neuroscience and psychology laboratory. *Inquiry, 52*(4), 378–398.

Bowen, C., Yeates, G., & Palmer, S. (2010). *A relational approach to rehabilitation: Thinking about relationships after brain injury*. London: Karnac Books.

Chen, T., Zhang, B., Deng, Y., Fan, J. C., Zhang, L., & Song, F. (2019). Long-term unmet needs after stroke: Systematic review of evidence from survey studies. *BMJ Open, 9*(5), 028137.

Coetzer, B. R., Vaughan, F. L., Roberts, C. B., & Rafal, R. (2003). The development of a holistic, community-based neurorehabilitation service in a rural area. *Journal of Cognitive Rehabilitation, 21*(1), 4–15.

Coetzer, R. (2014). Psychotherapy after acquired brain injury: Is less more? *Revista Chilena de Neuropsicología, 9*(1E), 36–41.

Coetzer, R., Evans-Roberts, C., Turnbull, O. H., & Vaughan, F. (2018). Neuropsychoanalytically-informed psychotherapy approaches to rehabilitation: The North Wales brain injury service – Bangor University experience 1998–2018. *Neuropsychoanalysis.* doi: 10.1080/15294145.2018.1478747

Couchman, G., McMahon, G., Kelly, A., & Ponsford, J. (2014). A new kind of normal: Qualitative accounts of multifamily group therapy for acquired brain injury. *Neuropsychological Rehabilitation, 24*(6), 809–832.

Downing, M., Hicks, A., Braaf, S., Myles, D., Gabbe, B., Cameron, P., . . . Ponsford, J. (2021). Factors facilitating recovery following severe traumatic brain injury: A qualitative study. *Neuropsychological Rehabilitation, 31*(6), 889–913.

Fleminger, S. (2008). Long-term psychiatric disorders after traumatic brain injury. *European Journal of Anaesthesiology, 25*(S42), 123–130.

Fraas, M. R., & Calvert, M. (2009). The use of narratives to identify characteristics leading to a productive life following acquired brain injury. *American Journal of Speech-Language Pathology, 18*(4), 315–328.

Glintborg, C., & Hansen, T. G. (2016). Bio-psycho-social effects of a coordinated neurorehabilitation programme: A naturalistic mixed methods study. *NeuroRehabilitation, 38*(2), 99–113.

Hammond, F. M., Barrett, R., Dijkers, M. P., Zanca, J. M., Horn, S. D., Smout, R. J., Guerrier, T., Hauser, E., & Dunning, M. R. (2015). Group therapy use and its impact on the outcomes of inpatient rehabilitation after traumatic brain injury: Data from traumatic brain injury-practice based evidence project. *Archives of Physical Medicine and Rehabilitation, 96*(8 Suppl), S282–S292.

Kreutzer, J. S., Seel, R. T., & Gourley, E. (2001). The prevalence and symptom rates of depression after traumatic brain injury: A comprehensive examination. *Brain Injury, 15*(7), 563–576.

Lexell, E. M., Alkhed, A. K., & Olsson, K. (2013). The group rehabilitation helped me adjust to a new life: Experiences shared by persons with an acquired brain injury. *Brain Injury, 27*(5), 529–537.

Lyon, I., Fisher, P., & Gracey, F. (2021). "Putting a new perspective on life": A qualitative grounded theory of posttraumatic growth following acquired brain injury. *Disability and Rehabilitation, 43*(22), 3225–3233.

Martin, D. J., Garske, J. P., & Davis, M. K. (2000). Relation of the therapeutic alliance with outcome and other variables: A meta-analytic review. *Journal of Consulting and Clinical Psychology, 68*(3), 438.

McDonald, S. (2017). Emotions are rising: The growing field of affect neuropsychology. *Journal of the International Neuropsychological Society, 23*(9–10), 719–731.

McKevitt, C., Fudge, N., Redfern, J., Sheldenkar, A., Crichton, S., Rudd, A. R., . . . Rothwell, P. M. (2011). Self-reported long-term needs after stroke. *Stroke, 42*(5), 1398–1403.

Newby, G., Coetzer, R., Daisley, A., & Weatherhead, S. (Eds.). (2013). *Practical neuropsychological rehabilitation in acquired brain injury. A guide for working clinicians.* London: Karnac Books.

Panksepp, J. (2004). *Affective neuroscience: The foundations of human and animal emotions.* Oxford: Oxford University Press.

Patterson, F., Fleming, J., & Doig, E. (2016). Group-based delivery of interventions in traumatic brain injury rehabilitation: A scoping review. *Disability and Rehabilitation, 38*(20), 1961–1986.

Ponsford, J. L., Downing, M. G., Olver, J., Ponsford, M., Acher, R., Carty, M., & Spitz, G. (2014). Longitudinal follow-up of patients with traumatic brain injury: outcome at two, five, and ten years post-injury. *Journal of Neurotrauma, 31*(1), 64–77.

Rao, V., & Lyketsos, C. (2000). Neuropsychiatric sequelae of traumatic brain injury. *Psychosomatics, 41*(2), 95–103.

Rohling, M. L., Faust, M. E., Beverly, B., & Demakis, G. (2009). Effectiveness of cognitive rehabilitation following acquired brain injury: A meta-analytic re-examination of Cicerone et al.'s (2000, 2005) systematic reviews. *Neuropsychology, 23*(1), 20–39.

Roth, A., & Fonagy, P. (2006). *What works for whom?: A critical review of psychotherapy research.* New York: Guilford.

Rowlands, L., Coetzer, R., & Turnbull, O. H. (2019). Good things better? Reappraisal and discrete emotions in ABI. *Neuropsychological Rehabilitation, 30*, 1947–1975. doi: 10.1080/09602011.2019.1620788.

Rowlands, L., Coetzer, R., & Turnbull, O. H. (2020). Building the bond: Predictors of the alliance in neurorehabilitation. *NeuroRehabilitation, 46*, 271–285. doi: 10.3233/NRE-193005.

Rowlands, L., Coetzer, R., & Turnbull, O. H. (2021). This time it's personal: Reappraisal after acquired brain injury. *Cognition and Emotion, 35*, 305–323. doi: 10.1080/02699931.2020.1839384.

Salas, C. E. (2012). Surviving catastrophic reaction after brain injury: The use of self-regulation and self-other regulation. *Neuropsychoanalysis, 14*(1), 77–92.

Salas, C. E., Casassus, M., Rowlands, L., Pimm, S., & Flanagan, D. A. (2018). "Relating through sameness": A qualitative study of friendship and social isolation in chronic traumatic brain injury. *Neuropsychological Rehabilitation, 28*(7), 1161–1178.

Salas, C. E., Gross, J. J., & Turnbull, O. H. (2019). Using the process model to understand emotion regulation changes after brain injury. *Psychology & Neuroscience, 12*(4), 430.

Salas, C. E., Turnbull, O. H., & Gross, J. J. (2014). Reappraisal generation after acquired brain damage: The role of laterality and cognitive control. *Frontiers in Psychology, 5*, 242.

Scholten, A. C., Haagsma, J. A., Cnossen, M. C., Olff, M., Van Beeck, E. F., & Polinder, S. (2016). Prevalence of and risk factors for anxiety and depressive disorders after traumatic brain injury: A systematic review. *Journal of Neurotrauma, 33*(22), 1969–1994.

Schultz, W., Dayan, P., & Montague, P. R. (1997). A neural substrate of prediction and reward. *Science, 275*(5306), 1593–1599.

Seligman, M. E. P. (2011). *Flourish: A visionary new understanding of happiness and well-being.* New York: Free Press.

Seligman, M. E. P., Steen, T. A., Park, N., & Peterson, C. (2005). Positive psychology progress: Empirical validation of interventions. *American Psychologist, 60*(5), 410–421.

Shotton, L., Simpson, J., & Smith, M. (2007). The experience of appraisal, coping and adaptive psychosocial adjustment following traumatic brain injury: A qualitative investigation. *Brain Injury, 21*(8), 857–869.

Tuckman, B. (1965). Developmental sequence in small groups. *Psychological Bulletin, 63*(6), 384–399.

Turner-Stokes, L., Pick, A., Nair, A., Disler, P. B., & Wade, D. T. (2015). Multi-disciplinary rehabilitation for acquired brain injury in adults of working age. *Cochrane Database of Systematic Reviews, 12.*

Walsh, M. E., Galvin, R., Loughnane, C., Macey, C., & Horgan, N. F. (2015). Community re-integration and long-term need in the first five years after stroke: Results from a national survey. *Disability and Rehabilitation, 37*(20), 1834–1838.

Wilson, B. A. (1997). Cognitive rehabilitation: How it is and how it might be. *Journal of the International Neuropsychological Society, 3*(5), 487–496.

Wilson, B. A., & Betteridge, S. (2019). The broad theoretical base of neuropsychological rehabilitation. In *Essentials of neuropsychological rehabilitation* (pp. 53–67). New York: Guilford Publications.

Wilson, B. A., & Gracey, F. (2009). Background and theory. Towards a comprehensive model of neuropsychological rehabilitation. In B. A. Wilson, F. Gracey, J. J. Evans, & A. Bateman (Eds.), *Neuropsychological rehabilitation: Theory, models, therapy and outcome* (pp. 1–22). Cambridge: Cambridge University Press.

11 Concrete patients need concrete therapists

Christian Salas

'Do not follow where the path may lead. Go instead where there is no path and leave a trail'.

—Ralph Waldo Emerson

1. Situation

I always warn trainees that clinical neuropsychology is a complex specialty, perhaps the most complex in clinical psychology. They often smile back at me, as if I am stating something obvious and irrelevant. But it is not until they start trying to help neurological patients to deal with their psychological suffering, and their psychosocial problems, that they really understand the meaning of my words. 'I can't work with this woman', commented a young trainee when supervising a patient with a right frontal stroke. 'She keeps talking and talking during sessions, as if she doesn't listen to a thing that I say!'. 'It's like he can't think', reported a deeply frustrated trainee working with a TBI survivor: 'He takes everything I say literally'. These are beautiful but painful moments in the formation of a clinical neuropsychologist. Beautiful because they can be a valuable opportunity to understand how brain damage can transform the mind: in thoughts and feelings, and in reconstructing identity. However, they can also be painful moments for the trainee, because therapists often feel deeply frustrated, powerless and even useless in these situations. Importantly, they can come to think that what they have been taught as clinical psychologists does not apply to 'organic' patients. As if patients with a brain injury belong to a different species,[1] or that they are only suitable for simplified versions of psychotherapy.

If we manage to steer these developmental crises in the right direction, situations like these can help trainees to refine their understanding of how brain injury alters the survivor's mentalising and relational abilities. This knowledge can also help trainees to really grasp how it 'feels' to be a mind-brain with a specific profile of neuropsychological impairments. Critically, it can also help them to see how others might experience this state from the outside.

I care about this problem because it tortured me for many years, and I found little guidance from colleagues and books. Some clinical psychologists,

DOI:10.4324/9781003300748-11

people I looked up to, told me it wasn't possible to work psychotherapeutically with this population. I remember one episode that marked me deeply. I was applying to a renowned postgraduate training programme in psychoanalytic psychotherapy. During the interview, I described the patients I was working with at that time, in a rehabilitation hospital: people with brain injuries that presented peculiar syndromes such as neglect, anosognosia, disinhibition or aphasia – all are very peculiar presenting features for a regular clinical psychologist. I remember that while I narrated my experience, I felt enthusiastic, not unlike a child that has found a rare and precious collecting card. I was expecting surprise and enthusiasm from my interviewers as well. I imagined the many opportunities that these patients opened for psychoanalysis, the many questions that could be explored regarding the mind and its biological substrate.[2] However, the memory of their response still hurts. One of them looked at me and said in a blasé tone: 'I don't know how we could help you with that here. I am not sure psychoanalysis can even be used with those patients'. Those patients? Of course, I did not make the cut for the programme. Thank God.

Along the years, I persevered with my belief that neurological patients could benefit from psychological interventions. Today, I know this is rather obvious, since there are many papers, and several books, on the topic (e.g. Klonoff, 2010; Ruff & Chester, 2014; Yeates & Ashworth, 2019). But back then there was little knowledge regarding how to implement those interventions, or how to adapt psychotherapeutic tools (Miller, 1993). Even more radical was the idea of using a psychoanalytic framework to work with these patients? Even more exotic and eccentric. The implicit belief at the time seemed to be that individuals with cognitive impairment needed behavioural and cognitive interventions. And that in order to use psychotherapeutic interventions with brain injury survivors, we should adapt its form and structure: notebooks to remember content from sessions, shorter sessions to avoid fatigue, use of a simple and straight-forward language, etc. (cf. Judd & Wilson, 2005). There was little consideration of how to help survivors to make sense of what happened to them, to generate meaning by supporting the mentalising process compromised by the injury, and to 'make the strange familiar'. Later I came to describe this as the problem of 'theoretical and technical adaptations'. Of course, patients with neurological impairments are extremely diverse, and the term 'brain damage' covers many diagnoses and presentations. So, the theoretical and technical adaptations needed are similarly diverse. However, changing the approach to individuals with concrete behaviour was my first laboratory. This is the story of how, from a single mistake and a single patient, everything started.

2. Example

Mr J was a 37-year-old man, who worked as a truck driver. He was married and had a young daughter. He had suffered a severe TBI after a car crash. As part of his in-patient rehabilitation programme, two hours of neuropsychology a week (therapy, from me) had been allocated by the physiatrist. Mr J was a tall and strong man, with no visible physical impairments, which was surprising considering the severity of his accident. During my routine interview he told me about his life as a truck driver, all the travelling it implied across the country, and how he learnt to drive trucks thanks to his father when he was quite young. I could tell by listening to Mr J's story that he loved his job, and was eager to leave the hospital, and resume his usual life. So far, so good. Mr J was also a pleasant man, always smiling, and cooperative throughout the interview. However, I began to sense something odd in our conversation. His answers tended to be brief, with no further elaboration. They were correct, but extremely succinct – typically just a few words. Indeed, I also gradually noticed that he never proposed a new topic, or took the conversation in another direction. He was always simply reactive to my questioning.

When I began asking about his accident, and the problems or changes it had generated in his life, I became even more concerned. According to Mr J, he was completely fine, and there were no problems at all. He recognised that his body was perhaps a little weak, but said this was improving with physiotherapy. And his mind? His mind was as sharp as usual, he replied. He also narrated this with a calm tone, and no sign of concern, even though he had been admitted to a rehabilitation unit. Interestingly, it also seemed that, for some reason, I started feeling restless and nervous when listening to him. How could I help him? I thought to myself. He believes he is perfectly fine. And to be honest, he looks happy, with no obvious signs of anxiety or depression.

After the first interview, every session was similar. He arrived on time and by himself. He was friendly, and appeared to really enjoy our time together. In fact, I did enjoy our sessions too. But bizarrely, he never brought a single complaint to a session. I caught myself, over and over again, trying to find something: a problem, a conflict, a sad feeling, to hold on to. With each passing session, I became more convinced there was something wrong with his communication – now I know what I witnessed is called Cognitive Communicative Disorder, which is extremely common after TBI. There was nothing wrong with his language, but he really struggled developing a fluid conversation and sharing information. Here is a transcription from a recording that I made.

CS: Hi J, how are you?
MR J: I am great dude . . .
CS: What's up?
MR J: super . . .
CS: How was your weekend?
MR J: fine . . .
CS: What did you do?
MR J: (15s) I did my homework . . .
CS: I see. But tell me something more. I imagine you did other things during the weekend.

MR J: yes, I visited my mom.

CS: Oh. Did you stay over?

MR J: yes . . .

CS: I see. And tell me, is your wife ok with you spending the night there?

MR J: yes . . . she doesn't complain.

CS: Really? She doesn't complain because you stay over the whole weekend, and she is on her own with your daughter?

MR J: no, not at all

I could see that something was amiss, and I imagined that a neuropsychological assessment could offer some clues. Clearly there was nothing wrong with his perception or language. His speed of processing was, however, slightly below average, and he struggled with digits backwards, or any task that required to manipulate information (like serial sevens: 100–7–7 . . .).

The more that I tried to assess executive functions, the more things fell apart. He completed the Trail Making Test A, but it took him over 3 minutes. And the B-version (with task switching) was an ordeal. He was more or less *never* able to alternate numbers and letters, and perseverated with the number sequence. Just like the text books. His performance on verbal fluency task was also really poor, offering on average three words for each letter, and long periods of silence. On the Similarities subtest, he struggled with simple items (shoes/socks: 'for your feet, to keep them warm'; ear/eyes: 'they are in your face'). Verbal memory was also compromised, particularly in the recollection phase. Overall, Mr J clearly presented a clear profile of executive impairment that much was clear. But he was not aware or concerned about these problems, nor the impact they might have in his life. For example, there was the real chance of his never returning to driving again.

A core feature of his presentation was the curious absence of 'other minds' in his narrative. At that time I used pictures of real life situations to explore patients' capacity to think about other people's mental states. One that I particularly liked showed a man and a woman sitting in front of a table. They were both loooking at something in front of them, something that could not be seen, but people often guessed it was a letter or an email. The woman's posture was informative: she supported her head with one hand while hugging the man with the other. She also had a Mona Lisa – like smile, which people often interpreted as a mixture of worry and sympathy. He did not show clear emotions in his face, but commonly people reported he was feeling concerned about the thing they were looking at. The instruction was simple and unstructured: 'Please describe what you see in this picture?'. If Mr J was not able to offer a suitable response, I would help him to focus on mental states, by asking 'Please tell me what you think she and he might be feeling or thinking?'.

If you try to picture in your mind my description of the scene, you may imagine a couple, perhaps dealing with financial difficulties? They look serious and perhaps upset. Or it might be some sort of discovery of an e-mail, that has undermined their relationship. Trying to imagine this scene, and the thoughts and feelings experienced by the characters in the picture, will help you to understand that human beings can be really abstract in their thinking. But people are typically not aware of this feature. Perhaps you are not aware of how readily we abstract? And perhaps *this* is why we struggle so much as clinicians when working with concrete patients.

Here is Mr J's response:

MR J: There is a guy writing in the computer . . . it seems. His hands are like that (imitates hands). There is also a girl hugging him (12s) that is it.

CS: What do you think might be going on between them? (the word *between* was my attempt to guide Mr J's attention to the relational space where the interaction takes place)

MR J: (13s) There is a guy writing, but I don't know what (16s).

CS: Look at the man on the right. Tell me what do you think he is thinking or feeling?

MR J: (21s) I can't imagine anything.

CS: What do you think she might be thinking or feeling?

MR J: . . . (50s)

CS: Any idea?

MR J: Yes, she might be thinking (58s). She might be having bad thoughts.

As with our interactions, and his performance on neuropsychological tests, Mr J was concrete in this mentalising task. He tended to focus on the visible features of the picture, neglecting what happened *between* the characters. Mental states are, of course, not always visible, and are often opaque. And people may feel something without showing it, or feel something completely different to what they show.

In addition, mental states are difficult to grasp because they may differ from our own, demanding that we inhibit our perspective to adopt someone else's perspective. Mr J struggled to go beyond what was obvious to the eyes, to dive into the subtleties of feelings and thoughts. Another way of describing Mr J's performance might be a lack of mental fluidity, an impairment in the generation of ideas. The main point here is that Mr J exhibited a concrete attitude towards the world, an attitude that compromised the capacity not only to reflect upon other people's mental states but also to access his own mental states, and connect with emotional experience and conflict.

3. Error

This takes us to the origin of my mistake. What role do we have, as clinical neuropsychologists, when our patients don't believe that they have problems? How do we help? Now I realise that patients like Mr J often make us feel insecure, and that insecurity makes us do things to recover a sense of usefulness. And so, to my eternal shame, I turned to cognitive training as a solution to my dilemma. I can clearly recall how, in that moment, I imagined that by retraining Mr J I would be useful again, that I had a purpose. That I had something I could show my colleagues and boss without embarrassment. Addressing the emotional situation of Mr J, helping him with his suffering, would have to wait. He was not ready yet, perhaps he was simply not feeling troubled by anything? He did not need any psychological support. So, I began the usual pen and paper cognitive drills during our sessions. Mr J took some of this work home. Indeed, he was extremely collaborative around the whole process.

Then came the bombshell. One day, Mr J arrived with his notebook, and while checking his homework I came across this:

Task: Write five things you do when you get up in the morning:

> Well, I get up and go to brush my teeth
> I get up and brush my teeth
> I get up and feed the dog
> I get up and go to take a shower
> Well, I get up and you will have to help me.

Task: Write five things you do before going to bed:

> Well, I get up and don't know what to do
> I get up and don't know what I would do
> I get up and don't know what to do
> Well, I have never fallen into despair
> Well, I have never . . ..

Reading Mr J's words was a striking moment of realisation for me – a realisation with several facets, all of which left me ashamed. It became suddenly clear to me that I had ignored Mr J's unawareness, and mistaken his inability to *speak* about his feelings as an absence of feelings themselves. Here was a man who was suffering, and I, his therapist, had failed to notice it because he could not verbalise it. That realisation hurt. Then there was the question of my choosing cognitive retraining. Here I was, attempting to re-train executive functions, when we know, when even *I* knew, that there is no credible evidence that this approach is effective.[3] Which invites the question of why I had chosen to ignore my own knowledge base? I provided the answer to this a few paragraphs ago: I felt unable to help him, and insecure, and I wanted to regain a sense of usefulness. In summary, the decision was a way to avoid negative counter-transferential feelings. Some moments of painful self-reflection followed.

In all of this complexity, the one mistake that still hurts, a mistake that is difficult to accept even today, is that I assumed there was no emotional experience underneath Mr J's placid exterior.

Had it not been for Mr J's 'homework', I might never have noticed. I could imagine Mr J at home, trying to complete the work I had prescribed. How he tries to think of something to write down, and yet a different idea interrupts his train of thought, leaving him unable to complete the task. Then a feeling emerges, perhaps of sadness or perplexity at his inability to think – a sadness that he is unable to escape from. In a sense, that feeling is the emotional equivalent of his performance on the Trail Making Test: the sadness persists, and in its perseveration, it captures his mind. He is sad, but he doesn't know why or what to do about it. He can't develop any ideas to downregulate the feeling, to change his actual situation[4]. Like a castaway that has been thrown into the sea, he holds onto anything he can grab: the thought of his therapist providing help, the thought of himself as someone that doesn't give up.

The dangerous mistake in this tale, which can be found even amongst professionals, is to think that brain injury survivors with cognitive impairment and unawareness have no emotional depth. By ignoring this, we dehumanise patients and under-value their sentience. We also break the first principle of neuropsychological rehabilitation: that the clinician must begin with patient's subjective experience, and work to reduce their frustration and confusion, in order to engage them in the rehabilitation process (Prigatano, 1999). In my defence, and perhaps in defence of other colleagues that have fallen into the same trap, the phenomenological experience of concrete patients is quite unique, and difficult to grasp for abstract neurotypical minds. This is why, as per the chapter title: concrete patients need concrete therapists (Salas et al., 2013). Therapists that are able to understand how the emotional landscape changes after the injury, and adapt their technical and theoretical tools to their needs and peculiarities.

4. Reflection

My mistake and initial encounter with the 'world of the concrete' sparked a series of questions about the phenomenological experience of patients like Mr J. Later I learnt that I was not the first to ask these questions. Kurt Goldstein and Martin Scherer (1941), for example, wrote an entire book trying to experimentally study abstract and concrete behaviour in patients with brain injury. In the famous Lanuti case, they described the impact that concreteness had on *all* cognitive domains, as well as emotional and social life (Hanfmann et al., 1944). I also discovered that what Goldstein called *concrete attitude* was similar to what modern authors have called the 'Default Mode', a realm of neural function that often re-emerges after frontal lobe lesions, where inflexible stimulus-response linkages remain impervious to modification by context or experience (Mesulam, 2002).

What the literature suggested was that Mr J's emotional experience was not abolished, but instead transformed. He appeared to have moments where emotions appeared that were related to grief, but they could not be re-activated in a therapeutic session. Somehow, Mr J was not able to do what many patients that attend psychotherapy do: they arrive telling the therapist that on a specific moment of the week something happened, and that they feel a certain way. Or they talk about how possible events from the future make them feel afraid or worried. Mr J was simply not able to bring his past emotional experiences to a session, nor activate emotional states based on future scenarios, because he was stuck in the present (Salas et al., 2013). We have called this difficulty generated by concreteness a change in the *temporal* dimension of the self. In addition, Mr J struggled to reflect upon his emotional and bodily states, or indeed upon *other* people's emotional states. Unlike many patients in psychotherapy, he struggled to detach from immediate experience when observing himself and others. We have called this difficulty a change in the *reflective* dimension of the self.

My mistake taught me that patients like Mr J *do* have emotional depth and conflicts. The problem was that I couldn't understand the logic of this view of the world. Due to my abstract mind, I was unable to grasp the peculiar world of the concrete, and how changes in the temporal and reflective dimension altered the emotional landscape. This understanding has ethical as well as clinical implications. The patient is grieving, but under the logic of the concrete. When we realise this, we cannot argue that concrete patients are not suitable for psychological interventions. We must acknowledge, instead, that most of our interventions are not *suitable* for these patients, and that we need to modify our interventions. Accordingly, we have proposed several modifications that can be incorporated to therapeutic work with these patients, in order to scaffold the temporal and reflective dimensions (Salas et al., 2013; Salas & Coetzer, 2015). Clinicians that work with concrete patients need to become familiar with the world of the concrete, and they need the flexibility to shift between concrete and abstract modes of functioning.

My journey trying to provide psychological interventions to patients with brain injury began with concrete patients. However, a similar logic can be applied to patients with other neuropsychological profiles. How do we work with an amnesic, or aphasic or impulsive patient?[5] We need to access their phenomenological field and understand how the specific profile of impairments changes his/her emotional landscape and mentalising capacities. Only by paying attention to the problem of theoretical and technical adaptations will we be able to provide the psychological care these patients need.

Notes

1 There are, strangely, still a few psychotherapists who hold this position (cf. Blass & Carmeli, 2007). For more on the barriers to working with brain injured patients, see Judd and Wilson (2005).

2 There is indeed an entire field, neuropsychoanalysis, which is dedicated to exactly this issue (see Solms & Turnbull, 2002, 2011; Salas et al., 2021).

3 There is a long history, since the middle of the last century (Luria, 1963), of neuropsychologists understanding that executive functions do not respond to the sort of training programmes that would for more basic cognitive skills.

4 We have since published a number of papers on this topic, some on the theme of the inability to self-regulate negative emotions after brain injury (Salas et al., 2013, 2014, 2015, 2019).

5 See Moore et al. (2017), Moore and Turnbull (2022) or Turnbull et al. (2006) for more on psychotherapy with profoundly amnesic patients. Or Kaplan-Solms and Solms (2000) or Salas et al. (2021) for therapeutic work with a range of other neuropsychological deficits, including those with aphasia.

References

Blass, R. B., & Carmeli, Z. V. I. (2007). The case against neuropsychoanalysis: On fallacies underlying psychoanalysis' latest scientific trend and its negative impact on psychoanalytic discourse. *The International Journal of Psychoanalysis, 88*(1), 19–40.

Goldstein, K., & Scheerer, M. (1941). Abstract and concrete behavior an experimental study with special tests. *Psychological Monographs, 53*(2), i.

Hanfmann, E., Rickers-Ovsiankna, M., & Goldstein, K. (1944). Case Lanuti: Extreme concretization of behavior due to damage of the brain cortex. *Psychological Monographs, 57*(4), i.

Judd, D., & Wilson, S. L. (2005). Psychotherapy with brain injury survivors: An investigation of the challenges encountered by clinicians and their modifications to therapeutic practice. *Brain Injury, 19*, 437–449. doi: 10.1080/02699050400010994

Kaplan-Solms, K., & Solms, M. (2000). *Clinical studies in neuro-psychoanalysis: Introduction to a depth neuropsychology* (2nd ed.). New York: Other Press.

Klonoff, P. S. (2010). *Psychotherapy after brain injury: Principles and techniques.* New York: Guilford Press.

Luria, A. R. (1963). *Restoration of function after brain injury.* Oxford: Pergamon Press.

Mesulam, M. M. (2002). *Principles of behavioral and cognitive neurology.* Oxford: Oxford University Press.

Miller, L. (1993). *Psychotherapy of the brain-injured patient: Reclaiming the shattered self.* New York: W. W. Norton & Co.

Moore, P. A., Dockree, S., Salas, C. E., & Turnbull, O. H. (2017). Observations on working psychoanalytically with a profoundly amnesic patient. *Frontiers in Psychology, 8*, 1418. doi: 10.3389/fpsyg.2017.01418

Moore, P. A., & Turnbull, O. H. (2022). Like a rolling stone: Psychotherapy without (episodic) memory. *Frontiers in Psychiatry, 13*, 958194. doi: 10.3389/fpsyt.2022.958194

Prigatano, G. P. (1999). *Principles of neuropsychological rehabilitation.* Oxford: Oxford University Press.

Ruff, R. M., & Chester, S. K. (2014). *Effective psychotherapy for individuals with brain injury.* New York: Guilford Publications.

Salas, C. E., & Coetzer, R. (2015). Is concreteness the invisible link between altered emotional processing, impaired awareness and mourning difficulties after traumatic brain injury? *Neuropsychoanalysis, 17*(1), 3–18.

Salas, C. E., Gross, J. J., Rafal, R., Viñas-Guasch, N., & Turnbull, O. H. (2013). Concrete behaviour and reappraisal deficits after a left frontal stroke: A case study. *Neuropsychological Rehabilitation, 23*, 467–500.

Salas, C. E., Gross, J. J., & Turnbull, O. H. (2014). Reappraisal generation after acquired brain damage: The role of laterality and cognitive control. *Frontiers in Emotion Science, 5*(242), 1–9. doi: 10.3389/fpsyg.2014.00242

Salas, C. E., Gross, J. J., & Turnbull, O. H. (2019). Using the process model to understand emotion regulation changes after brain injury. *Psychology and Neuroscience, 12*, 430–450. http://dx.doi.org/10.1037/pne0000174

Salas, C. E., Turnbull, O. H., & Solms, M. (Eds.). (2021). *Clinical studies in neuropsychoanalysis revisited.* New York: Routledge.

Salas, C. E., Vaughan, F., Shanker, S., & Turnbull, O. H. (2013). Stuck in a moment, Concreteness and psychotherapy after acquired brain injury. *Journal of Neuro-disability & Psychotherapy, 1*(1), 1–38.

Solms, M., & Turnbull, O. H. (2002). *The brain and the inner world: An introduction to the neuroscience of subjective experience.* New York: Other Press.

Solms, M., & Turnbull, O. H. (2011). What is neuropsychoanalysis? *Neuropsychoanalysis*, *2*, 133–145.

Turnbull, O. H., Zois, E., Kaplan-Solms, K., & Solms, M. (2006). The developing transference in amnesia: Changes in inter-personal relationship despite profound episodic memory loss. *Neuropsychoanalysis*, *8*, 199–204.

Yeates, G. N., & Ashworth, F. (Eds.). (2019). *Psychological therapies in acquired brain injury*. New York: Routledge.

12 It's getting worse, Doc.

Rudi Coetzer

'No man is an island entire of itself'.

—John Donne

1. Situation

Clinical neuropsychologists who work in community settings are often able to follow up their patients long-term. As a result, they may get to know the people they see quite well over time. But how well? For example, we might become more certain about their diagnoses, its likely severity, and the impairments from their brain injury. Clinical neuropsychologists, also with time, learn quite a bit more about how a specific person's difficulties manifest out there in the 'real' world. We learn that each brain injury is different, even if they seem superficially similar. For example, two individuals may have sustained remarkably similar traumatic brain injuries, at least as regards clinical markers of severity, and even also the distribution of contusions on scan. But these two persons may well present quite differently in the clinic, and especially in everyday life. These differences depend, of course, on several factors, including premorbid personality, family support and their broader socio-economic setting. I sometimes wonder whether we are all born with similar hardware, but over time a different combination of software is installed for each of us.

There is also time since injury, which determines presentations, and trajectories of change after acquired brain injury. I'd heard it argued that time is the greatest healer. But time equally is also a great teacher. Let's elaborate a little, by taking a hypothetical case of a person with a severe traumatic brain injury, sustained six months earlier. The clinical neuropsychologist, working in an outpatient setting, starts seeing them at this point. Let's say baseline neuropsychological testing is performed at about nine months post-injury. Then this patient enters rehabilitation, accessing various therapies, including (amongst several others) group-based interventions. This in turn is followed by some individual psychological work, for example cognitive behaviour therapy to help with anxiety, and encourage more sustained levels of participation in social and leisure activities. After this phase, the clinical neuropsychologist, service configuration permitting, may wish to periodically review and 'problem shoot'

DOI:10.4324/9781003300748-12

with the patient. By now it is a good three to four years post-injury. Are things getting better, or at least remaining the same? Or has time not been such a great healer and made things worse?

2. Situation

Huw was in his late 50s when he sustained a moderate traumatic brain injury after falling, while out climbing in the mountains. On the morning when he fell, Huw was with other climbers, who managed to phone the emergency services. His fellow climbers administered first aid, for what looked like a fractured left leg. Their main concern was that Huw remained unconscious, but at least he was breathing unaided. After a few hours, he was airlifted by the mountain rescue team to the nearest acute care hospital, where a CT scan of the brain revealed the presence of small bilateral frontal and temporal contusions. X-rays confirmed that he had fractured his leg. Huw was admitted to ITU, and regained consciousness later that evening, in as much as that he was awake, although quite passive. The next day he was transferred to an orthopaedic ward. Here Huw remained for a further ten days. Huw posed no problems to staff, and presented with no behavioural difficulties. He received physiotherapy while an inpatient, and was discharged home after a total length of stay in hospital of 12 days. He received a few home visits from a community physiotherapist to help him with his mobility.

On initial assessment, three months post-injury, Huw came to the attention of the community brain injury service. He presented with very few complaints himself, but did volunteer that he *might* have a poor memory, though he 'did not really think so'. When asked what that meant, he said that while he actually thought he had a good memory his wife, Sioned, had noticed that he often forgot appointments. Actually, he said that he 'allegedly' forgot appointments . . . or items on a shopping list, or household chores. Sioned, immediately listed a few examples of Huw forgetting to do things. He laughed about her comments regarding his memory problems. Actually, he said, there were hardly any memory problems – or nothing too problematic. For example, he could remember everything back to even his primary school days! And anyway, he was sure that most people would sometimes forget things.

The GP, on the other hand, who made the referral, said that Huw had made a good recovery, and had no obvious cognitive problems. From the GP's point of view, the main concern was really that Huw was much less engaged in activities than he had been. The nature of this apathy extended to even include mountaineering, which he used to love. Now that his leg has been rehabilitated, and his mobility back to normal, why would that be? Perhaps Huw was anxious? When presented with this, Huw was a bit perplexed about the anxiety hypothesis. He remembered nothing about the episode on the mountain, and from his perspective had no anxiety about climbing. Instead, his main problem, he said, was that he just could not be *bothered* to climb, because he had 'new interests'. But when asked, he could not list a single one of these new interests.

Was Huw perhaps depressed? He did seem a bit lacking in energy and drive. Maybe that was obscuring an unhappiness that was not immediately apparent. That could explain why he was not the most talkative, unless actively engaged in conversation by another person. But on the other hand, Huw *was* able to express positive affect. He just was not that *interested* in doing things. In fact, he reported that when he *was* taken to say an outing or other activity, once engaged in what was happening, he actually enjoyed it.

Moreover, Huw had no biological markers of depression. He was sleeping well, his appetite was good and he had lost no weight over the past couple of months. Huw also retained a good sense of future, and talked quite freely about the many plans he had for different projects, now that he had more time on his hands. The only problem was that he never *acted* upon these plans. Sioned, his wife, found this difficult, and said it was pointless to ask him to do any chores now. Unsurprisingly then, one of our early rehabilitation interventions was to get Huw to exercise more regularly. Through a national hospital exercise referral scheme, Huw was provided with a place at a local gym, to attend twice a week over a period of three months. Transport was arranged to take him to the gym, and he reported enjoying going there. At the end of the three months however, he did not join the gym, and never returned.

It was the same story with other activities the occupational therapist arranged for him. Provided all the scaffolding was in place, Huw would attend, and by all accounts enjoy whatever activity it was he went to. He particularly liked the woodwork classes, and said that 'the blokes there were good lads'. But unless he was taken by hospital transport, he made no effort to go to these sessions, and seemed quite unconcerned about missing sessions. Huw also went to the service's psycho-education groups, and successfully completed the block of ten sessions. He told his therapists that he 'learned a lot about the brain', and that it was 'a fascinating course'.

What of this other problems? Huw had recovered well from his fractured leg, and did not require ongoing physiotherapy. There were no speech or language difficulties, and he was not seen by the team's speech therapist. As part of his individual neuropsychology sessions, Huw was offered psychological therapy, which he did not engage with. He also was given a comprehensive baseline neuropsychological testing, to determine his relative cognitive strengths and vulnerabilities. This was completed at roughly one-year post-injury.

Huw's baseline neuropsychological testing revealed a complex set of results. He showed good effort throughout the testing, and did not experience any obvious fatigue. As for premorbid function, he scored within the 'above average' range, which was also consistent with his Wechsler Adult Intelligence Scale scores. Indeed, the latter also showed very little difference between the respective Index Scores. In the round, Huw's language functions were all also within the expected range for his own premorbid abilities. However, his processing speed was one and a half standard deviation below what would have been expected for him. Similarly, as regards memory functions, auditory learning and recall were a standard deviation below the expected, and visual learning and recall one and a half standard deviations below.

The most striking impairments though were in the domain of executive control. Huw performed nearly three standard deviations below his expected on the Wisconsin Card Sorting Test, and failed to complete the Tower of Hanoi. It was also very noticeable that he had a poor organisational strategy when copying the Rey Complex Figure. Undoubtedly, his initial poor planning and organisation also adversely affected his delayed recall of the figure. Overall, the protocol appeared compatible with the expected effects of a TBI. Furthermore, to a fair degree his cognitive profile matched the feedback Sioned provided regarding her husband's functioning out 'in the real world'.

As part of his cognitive rehabilitation, Huw was helped with some memory compensatory strategies, as well as some routines and strategies to improve planning and organisation skills. These mostly centred on Huw making use of his phone's calendar and reminder functions, as well as using a notepad for phone messages at home. Admittedly, it did take him a bit of time and practice to learn to *always* leave the notebook on the little table by the telephone; otherwise, he would regularly forget to take down messages and numbers of callers. Huw gradually became more settled in his new routines, which one might also describe as his pattern of lack of engagement in regular activities. This remained a big bugbear to Sioned. But despite this, Huw seemed happy in himself, and content with how things were. It also appeared as if Sioned, while not particularly pleased with his lack of involvement, was tolerating the situation fairly well. She certainly did not report that it was causing major problems, so it was sensible to avoid digging where there are no obvious problems. With this in mind, Huw went onto our system of long-term care, meaning he would be seen every six months for a clinical review. The main purpose of these sessions was really to determine if there were any changes in his clinical presentation, to some extent representing a relapse prevention mechanism. We had reached a position of stability, even if the situation wasn't ideal.

At around three years post-injury, Huw came back to clinic for repeat neuropsychological testing, in response to a personal injury insurance claim on a policy he owned coming to a close. Assessment would also help to determine his progress since the baseline testing almost two years ago. Huw performed similarly relative to baseline, except that his auditory learning and recall was improved to approximately half a z-score above that of a year earlier, and his visual learning and recall improved to the same magnitude. The rest of the test profile was almost identical to baseline. Huw seemed pleased with the feedback that his memory had improved. He wondered if his keeping of lists was helping him remember things, and said that he was 'doing well'. On further probing, it again transpired that he was certainly happy in himself, but not really engaging with regular, meaningful activities. Alas, Sioned failed to attend this appointment, so there was no collateral feedback about his actual functioning in the community. Nevertheless, we agreed that given that he seemed quite settled, he should now come back to clinic annually, or as needed in between by self-referral. Huw was happy with this plan of action.

Huw diligently attended his annual reviews over the next five years – always on time, almost as if delivered by an external force. His presentation did not change, and he was really easy to manage in terms of clinical review and relapse prevention. His wife attended one or two of the earlier reviews, but presented as quite disengaged. Sioned mentioned that she had returned to work as an academic, and that she was expected to travel as part of her role. There was clear sadness to be detected in her description of how her role in the marriage had changed, and that she felt lonely and isolated. She reflected that perhaps going back to work might help. She was encouraged to access the service's relatives support group, but did not take this up. In fact, Sioned never attended any appointments with Huw again. At subsequent review meetings Huw said she was very busy with her work, and that she sent her apologies for not attending. Huw nevertheless continued to present in almost exactly the same way. He was not using the four-wheel drive vehicle he bought with some of the money from the pay-out of his personal injury policy, despite his plans to 'get out into nature a bit more', and go camping in remote areas. He had all the gear, but no plans nor intentions to actually use it.

Then one day there was a message from Huw. He felt he needed to come to clinic for review. Seven months early. Because this was highly unusual for Huw, he was offered the very next cancellation. As was now the usual routine, he attended on his own. However, something was wrong. Maybe he gained a bit of weight? But that would be expected, given how inactive he had been the past decade or so. He also looked tired? Maybe he had a bad night's sleep? Or perhaps he was just getting a bit older, and showing his age due to not exercising regularly. Huw though thought none of these were of concern. His main worry was that he was 'getting worse'. Why would that be? He had no idea. But Huw said to me that it was obvious his memory was much worse, and getting 'poorer by the week'. That would, of course, run counter to research findings relating to the trajectory of cognition over time after traumatic brain injury, and Huw was duly reassured that he 'was probably now just a bit more aware of his memory difficulties', than say five or so years ago. However, Huw then dropped the bombshell. He also recently started experiencing unilateral throbbing headaches. And to top it all, they were associated with photophobia and nausea. In response Huw was reviewed by the team's neurologist.

The neurologist's verdict was that Huw's headaches were the result of taking too many painkillers, so that he had developed rebound headaches. The neurologist also pointed out that most headaches are benign, and that in any case, a substantial proportion of patients with traumatic brain injury experience headaches. It seemed that there was nothing ominous going on, and certainly nothing like, for example, a brain tumour. He was, the neurologist said, simply to stop taking his over-the-counter analgesic medication so regularly. However, Huw previously denied over-using regular painkillers. The neurologist thought maybe something else might be at play, and sent Huw back for further neuropsychology input.

At the neuropsychology review Huw said he started taking some painkillers to help him at night, codeine put him to sleep, but then it had stopped being effective. As a result, he had to take more, but he denied that it was excessive use. But what is excessive? Could we have a trial reduction? Even after stopping his painkillers for a month, he was still complaining of 'horrendous memory problems', and that it was 'definitely getting worse'. There was only one way to find out more about this. Huw would need to be re-assessed. He seemed pleased with this. He did not mind this, and indeed it would be the fourth time (he was also one tested by a colleague in private practice for the insurance company).

When Huw's fourth neuropsychological testing was completed and scored up, he was invited in for feedback. He failed to attend (one of those DNA – Did not attends) but made the next one offered. Huw was given the good news. His memory was not deteriorating at all. In fact, he had improved even more. Not a lot, but all previous memory scores were now either at the same level or about one quarter of a z score up. This was good news – very good news. Except that Huw did not look pleased. Rather, he looked shattered, or more accurately, tired, sad, and exhausted. What on earth was going on? Most patients are relieved when they are reassured about their memory, and in particular when they hear that they are not deteriorating, but perhaps have just become more aware of their memory lapses.

Did this positive news match his experience? No. He reported forgetting to do chores, the house was in chaos. Really? Was Sioned not writing his daily chores on the whiteboard in the kitchen anymore? Huw started to cry. Sioned had left him four months ago. Actually, he said, he had seen very little of her the previous five months anyway. Her work now consumed all her energies. Actually, he finally reported, he thought she had met someone else. Whatever the case, she had made it clear that she was not returning. Everything was falling apart for Huw, and my patient had lost the one person who had been maintaining a sense of coherence in his life.

3. Error

There are two broad areas of erroneous clinical reasoning illustrated in this case. The first concerns retesting. While it is good practice to perform retesting of some (but not all) patients, the clinical neuropsychologist should always keep the specific indications for re-testing clear in mind. In particular the question: Why now, in this person's case, am I retesting. Is it to map the trajectory of recovery and rehabilitation gains? Or is it a condition with a likelihood of cognitive decline? Has there been a change in clinical presentation suggesting an additional neurological disorder?

Whatever the indications might be, determining whether test scores have actually, reliably, changed, is a complex process. And influenced by many factors, most notably practice effects, and using parallel forms (Duff, 2012). These should give every neuropsychologist pause for thought. If only *these* two factors (never mind age norms, and clinical versus statistical significance) are considered, modestly 'improved' scores may actually mean no change. They may even, depending on magnitude, reflect a slight decrease. It is essential that clinical neuropsychologists carefully consider changes in test scores, given that the conclusions and feedback may have a real impact on patients and their relatives.

The second area of poor clinical reasoning concerns the failure to spot psychosocial stressors, gradually coming into play over time. Looking back over the evolution of Huw's care and review, it should now be clear how, due to his apathy or lack of engagement, his wife became more and more disengaged, and finally drifted away. Alas, all too common a story after TBI. I had failed to spot, or at least more closely consider *why* Huw's wife was not attending review sessions anymore. Who knows whether, with earlier detection and intervention, Huw's marital breakdown could potentially have been avoided, through for example couples therapy, or more robust behavioural interventions to get Huw a bit more engaged? The essential point is that I failed to continually fine tune the formulation, by obtaining small but important collateral feedback from those living with the patient. Patients are often able 'to keep the show on the road', or put on a brave face, during a relatively short clinical review appointment. You have time with them, but alas all too often they fail to report ongoing concerns, they minimise their problems, or may even (perhaps due to poor self-awareness?) deny that they have problems at home or work. It can be critically important to get a genuine report from what might otherwise seem like a routine annual review.

4. Reflection

While it is a privilege for the clinical neuropsychologist to be able to provide long-term follow-up to their patients, we should guard against complacency, especially with 'easy' patients, where things seem settled and unchanged over several years.

This might be read as a request to regularly review and update hypotheses. However, this might not be enough. The astute clinical neuropsychologist should also consider *new* hypotheses. In particular non-biological ones, because our patients are people with lives outside of the hospital, including life events affecting them, which may have no relation to their history of a brain injury.

Importantly, while these life events are not necessarily biological in nature, some are very interweaved with the brain injury and its effect. Not infrequently manifesting on a systemic (e.g. family or work level) rather than intra-individual level. In some cases, it would be essential to work more systematically during brain injury rehabilitation, and closely involve a spouse, or the family as a whole, to secure better outcomes (Bowen, 2007) for patients. Maybe realising within the old tried and tested biopsychosocial model, that within neuropsychological formulations, things evolve over time, and with increased time, biological factors might dominate less than we think. Yes, things can get worse many years after acquired brain injury, but not always for the reasons we think.

References

Bowen, C. (2007). Family therapy and neuro-rehabilitation: Forging a link. *International Journal of Rehabilitation and Therapy*, 14 (8): 344–349.
Duff, K. (2012). Evidence-based indicators of neuropsychological change in the individual patient: Relevant concepts and methods. *Archives of Clinical Neuropsychology*, 27: 248–261.

13 Not built in a day

Rudi Coetzer

'Success does not consist in never making mistakes, but in never making the same one a second time'.

—George Bernard Shaw

1. Situation

Browsing through the neuropsychological rehabilitation research literature and various textbooks, one would swear that six (or eight, or is it now 12?) sessions of Cognitive Behaviour Therapy (CBT) can 'cure' any presenting problem (or combination of problems) after acquired brain injury (for example, Department of Health, 2005). Perhaps this is an unfair generalisation – not least because CBT is actually a good evidence-based psychological therapy for many of our patients. However, there is some truth in the fact that clinical neuropsychologists are expected, by those less in the know, to 'make things better'. The main issue is not only that things should get *better*, but also that it is more the expectation of delivering a 'cure', within the time constraints of funding, deadlines, reports or relatives' wishes, and so on. No wonder that many clinical neuropsychologists working in rehabilitation settings early on in their careers, develop a sense of urgency that they 'must do something to fix a problem'.

Working in multi-professional teams sometimes further potentiates this belief amongst us. Everybody else seems to have an 'episode of care', or 'treatment block' which they deliver to their patients, and with clear endpoints. The physiotherapist provides tangible treatments, with clear outcomes, the occupational therapist helps the patient to re-learn crucial skills (and gets them home . . .), and the doctor prescribes medication for well-defined symptoms. But the 'talking cure', where does that fit in? Sometimes, actually rather often, the actual goals of psychological therapy are too vague. Speaking to practicing colleagues, there is frequent allusion to expectations outweighing what can realistically be achieved. 'Are you *still* seeing that patient? I thought she had been discharged long ago?'

2. Example

The thing about Tom is how big he was. Really big. A powerfully built man in his mid-40s, complete with number one haircut, ferocious tattoos, and a

DOI:10.4324/9781003300748-13

'one size too small t-shirt'. Tom had sustained a severe traumatic brain injury two decades previously. At the time there was very little rehabilitation available, other than that for his physical difficulties with fine motor control. Physically Tom made a reasonably good recovery. However, he presented with very significant cognitive impairment, poor emotional regulation – most pressing of all, with behavioural difficulties. It was for the latter that his general practitioner referred him for 'psychological help with his personality problems after a very serious head injury years ago'. Tom was discussed and allocated during a weekly multi-professional team meeting. As was normally the case, his referral was considered along with many others referred for neuropsychological testing, rehabilitation, or other interventions. My first encounter with Tom was when he attended for his first appointment in clinic.

Reassuringly I had done my 'homework'. That is, trawled his bundle, or put differently, read over all of his medical records prior to his attendance. In theory, the purpose of this is to obtain as much as possible of a patient's history before they attend. It is considered good practice to familiarise oneself with a referral, avoiding unnecessary questions about what is already known. Naturally, it is also crucial to confirm the actual evidence for say a traumatic brain injury or stroke, rather than just blindly take at face value what is contained in a referral letter. Furthermore, there is also some suggestion that it is good for the therapeutic relationship if patients can see that clinician has taken an interest in their case. It helps to have done some work before the first meeting. One can also do background work for developing a rehabilitation plan or strategy.

The plan for the first session was to look more closely at what specific behaviours were of concern to Tom, checking where, when and under what circumstances these occurred. Once I had a better understanding of the specifics of his presenting problems, I would offer Tom a treatment plan, most likely consisting of goal setting, CBT and behavioural activation. Of crucial importance also, was to 'contract'. We would set some specific goals together, specify how many psychological therapy sessions before reviewing progress, and at which frequency (typically once a week). This was the 'block' of therapy. Outcome measurement would consist of comparing post-intervention questionnaires, and rating scale scores with baseline data. That was, at least in theory, how clinical neuropsychologists offer tangible, measurable, rehabilitation interventions.

But Tom was having none of my well-prepared plan. Things started badly when he did not quite understand what all the questions were about. He asked me several times to repeat myself. He got more and more annoyed. Before too long, Tom started shouting and swearing. I worked even harder at trying to explain to him what we needed to do, in order to help him. But every sentence seemed to make things worse, only serving to turn up the temperature in the room yet another degree. The situation became much worse when, after about an hour, I indicated that our time for today was up. Indeed, reflecting quietly by myself, the first of the ten sessions were up. Tom shouted at me that I had no time for him, and that I was running off to see people who had 'no problems, were only alcoholics'. I had no idea what this was about, but decided it would be unwise to ask. At least there were nine sessions left to right the situation.

The next session did not go well either. Being a couple of minutes late was a felony from Tom's perspective. I attempted to defuse the situation, trying to explain why I was two minutes late . . . as well as the relative scale of two minutes in the greater scheme of 24 hours of each day. That was a mistake. Tom got so angry that I thought he might have a heart attack. His failure to grasp what seemed so obvious to others was beginning to create a very significant barrier to engagement with psychological therapy.

This was a great pity, because in the first session I had developed a good psychological therapy plan, for helping him manage his obviously problematic behaviours, which in turn surely were fuelled by inaccurate cognitions. Well, nothing like the here and now, in-session behaviours, to serve as real examples that should prove fertile ground for explaining the rationale for CBT. I said to Tom that we should look at his thoughts, behaviours and feelings and see how these differ, but influence each other. There was the shortest of silences, before he stormed out, the echoes of profanities following him down the corridor, before disappearing out of the front door of the clinic.

Session three? Well, what can one say? Tom attended, I was on time, but nothing happened. Mid-way through the session, I found myself wondering if metaphorically we spoke different languages. While we both spoke English, we could not understand each other. I was a bit more careful with explaining the rationale of CBT. . . . At some point when Tom started to become irritated, I suggested we look at what he was thinking? The suggestion appeared to stop him in his tracks, so I quickly followed up with a simplified explanation of how our thoughts influence how we feel. And what we do. And indeed what we *don't* do. He looked at me, stunned, as if I had switched to German mid-sentence. Keeping things light, I said that: 'It's really simple: what we think and how we experience certain emotions make us behave in certain ways. And for this reason, I was wondering what he was thinking when he was feeling irritated. The rest of the session was a torrent of irritation, agitation and swearing, mostly consisting of examples of interpersonal conflict that he was experiencing out in the community.

At the weekly multi-professional team meeting our physiotherapist asked how I was getting on with Tom, she noticed that he was religiously attending his sessions with me. Also that by the way, he was progressing with his exercise. He liked weight training. Feeling my face go red while the team's attention was now turned towards me for my feedback, I waffled something about trying to form a therapeutic relationship. The physiotherapist asked me how many sessions I was going to see him for, as she had another psychotherapy referral for me. I asked her to hang on just a little bit. I said I was actually floundering with Tom, but felt it was too early to end the sessions. There was something that was odd. Why was he continuing to attend if therapy was such a miserable failure? Why, despite the fact that we appeared to be at loggerheads for most of the session? Why were we unable to understand what we were trying to say to each other? Maybe I should give him homework, stuff to read, to accelerate his acquisition of the basic principles underpinning CBT?

Our next session started well. I asked Tom how he was, and then kept my mouth shut. He talked and tried to tell me . . . something. It was unclear what was on Tom's mind. He struggled to string sentences together, struggled to find words and frequently forgot what he was trying to convey. But he seemed calm enough, which made a welcome change. Three quarters through the session I started to worry that I was paid way too much to be sitting here doing nothing. There were only six appointments left, and we have made no progress yet. Was the best I could come up with, simple listening, or basic counselling (Rogers, 1961)? Surely that was not enough, and certainly not what was expected from an experienced clinical neuropsychologist who has worked in several different healthcare settings, including the NHS. So, without further ado, I told Tom that I had some stuff for him to read in preparation of our next session. He stuffed the reading material into a jacket pocket and asked when I would be seeing him again. We were, I thought, finally making progress.

Tom was very annoyed from the word go during our next session. The ambulance transport was late picking him up, so he arrived a few minutes late for his appointment. Don't worry about it, I will still see you, I patiently explained trying to reassure him. That did not go down with Tom at all. He shouted that he would go private. Money was no option. Fuelled by an instantaneous bout of severe counter-transference, I pointed out some recent findings about state healthcare (the NHS), versus the independent sector, no actually, the supposed best hospitals in world – America. And that there would be no evidence to support his belief that he would get better care elsewhere than at a service such as ours, anywhere in the world. The only difference would be that he would have to pay for something he can access for free, like millions of others, which was a very unwise strategy. . . . Clearly counter transference got the better of me. Tom went red in his face, reached into his pocket, grabbed a handful of coins and flung these across the room. Together we had managed to press not only the counter-transference switch but also the transference nuclear launch button. Strangely though, Tom left the session in fairly good spirits a few minutes later. How intriguing.

Yes, of course Tom had many of the classic impairments associated with severe traumatic brain injury. He had poor self-awareness, was repetitive, struggled to remember what was said from the one minute to the next, and had real problems with emotion regulation. I was very aware of these, and in particular how they explained and influenced his presentation. However, it did not quite capture the ferocity of what was happening in the consultation room. Furthermore, his impairments and brain scan findings of frontal and temporal contusions were entirely compatible with severe traumatic brain injury. But there was more to it. Why were we getting nowhere in psychotherapy? Was psychotherapy a waste of time? Maybe, or, perhaps maybe for Tom. Time was running out, and the waiting list was, well . . . waiting. My colleagues on the other hand were (mostly) achieving their goals and outcomes, patients were improving as regards walking, making a cup of tea, and with not that many sessions required either. Another visceral I-am-paid-too-much crisis moment was upon me before I could . . . think.

During the second half of Tom's sessions a few things happened. Increasingly I started feeling a sense of dread when I saw in the clinic schedule that he was due to see me on the day. His agitation and irritability almost inevitably spilled over into frank aggression. Moreover, it was almost always in response to what appeared like a totally insignificant event during the session. For example, not quite hearing or understanding what he was saying (Tom had dysarthria) – or saying the wrong thing, interrupting, or looking at him 'funny'. The sessions, in his view, ended too soon. It all felt too much like continual dance away from an overwhelmingly stronger opponent during a sports contest, to stay out of harm's way. Like a fullback doing a locum in the scrum. I had an overwhelming sense that neither of us enjoyed these sessions, and if we were more honest, we would have chosen to end the endeavour straight away. By the end of most of his sessions, Tom looked more agitated than when we arrived. Effectively, my intervention made him feel worse than he was prior to attendance. I was often convinced he would not show for his next appointment.

But Tom kept on coming back. I was becoming more perplexed. Why would he continue to attend his appointments with me if the therapeutic relationship was so poor? I needed all the help I could get. However, discussing these themes during supervision shed no further light on the situation. My supervisor looked stumped too. The plan was sound, but clearly not working. The only advice from my supervisor was to prevent conflict and keep on chipping away at forging the therapeutic relationship. Which, to my defence, was of course exactly what I have been trying to do. Gradually something started to dawn on me. Maybe on this occasion I have failed to help my patient. It is important for clinicians to be open to their failures and take appropriate actions. A niggling thought started to enter my mind, which was to 'do the right thing' and discharge him. There were no alternatives. None of my colleagues had any enthusiasm for taking over Tom's care from me. They had seen enough during his brief periods in our waiting room. At least the 'contracted' ten sessions were rapidly coming to an end. Might there be at least some solace in the thought that 'I had delivered what was contracted'?

During one of my supervision sessions, I decided to grasp the nettle. What if we (me) simply cannot form a therapeutic relationship with a patient (in this case Tom)? My supervisor and I reflected on several possible reasons. Maybe my technique was wrong – should I consider using another psychotherapeutic model? CBT is not for everyone. Or sometimes we just cannot engage a given patient, in which case the right thing might well be to discharge or refer to a colleague for a second attempt. None of these suggestions were new, and in fact had been at the forefront of my own thinking about how to manage the situation. In reality, the nature of Tom's sessions by now had made me realise that we were never going to 'hook' him to listen to how his thoughts were central to his problems, never mind practice techniques how to change them! I pointed out to my supervisor that I had long ago retreated to the safe side-lines of Rogerian reflections (Rogers, 1961). Or just kept quiet and tried to come across as empathic and non-threatening. Thinking about it though, this did seem to at least reduce his agitation. But I had clearly failed to 'make things better'.

Tom and I met for our last session. He looked fine with the fact that it was the last time he would be seeing me. And I decided it was probably best to let sleeping dogs lie. An increasingly familiar pattern commenced. Tom laboriously strung together what was bothering him this week, often failing to find the words, or remember what he was actually talking about. I tried an interpretation that perhaps his behaviour might have something to do with the interpersonal conflict he experiences so regularly. And that maybe this was a factor contributing to his social isolation. Tom went ballistic. But it did not matter, as his therapy was anyway ending – there was no point in today following the usual approach of trying to point out to him the 'error of his ways'. I kept my mouth shut, and looked out of the window, trying to remember who else I was seeing over the course of the remainder of the afternoon. Tom's tirade was continuing in the background, creating its own din of dissatisfaction. There's a limit to what even the most experienced therapist can absorb.

Despite racking my memory, I could not for the life of me recall who was coming to see me later that afternoon. Just a void, and unusual for me not to remember my clinic schedule. But then I became aware of something else which was unusual. What's wrong with the room? It's gone all quiet. I looked back from staring out of the window and noticed that Tom was looking at me. I spontaneously commented that he looked a bit more relaxed. Tom pondered this for a minute or two, before saying that 'it feels good to talk'. The remainder of the session I said very little. When the session ended, we walked towards reception. Unexpectedly, Tom asked me how I was. A bit stunned, I replied that I was well, thank you, and that it was nice of him to ask. Tom beamed, and for a brief moment looked, well . . . just like a normal person. I felt a sense of sorrow, and guilt. The poor man. It must be so difficult for him. For the first time, I had a brief sense of just how awful things must be for him. Before he left, Tom asked his usual question of when he will receive his next appointment letter. He has obviously forgotten that his block of ten sessions for psychological therapy ended today. And that was that.

3. Errors

With the benefit of hindsight, it should be possible for most readers to identify several errors made by the clinician (me) responsible for Tom's psychological therapy. For example, while preparing rehabilitation, or psychological therapy, we should plan in advance, though the plan should never be rigidly stuck to. Furthermore, sticking to one therapeutic model, come what may, is often not a good approach either. In passing, and of note, there were clearly issues for me with managing the counter-transference.

But the main error relates to time. The focus on, and tensions around a time-limited episode of care, followed by planned discharge, is the most obvious symptom of this error. What exactly underpinned the decision to provide ten sessions of CBT? The research literature? Textbooks? And how does that align with working with a condition which is acknowledged to result in chronic impairments associated with long-term disability?

In the UK, the National Service Framework for Long Term Neurological Conditions (2005) recognises that patients should be seen long-term for psychological input. This is of course entirely sensible. Acquired brain injury more often than not results in a suite of cognitive impairment, poor self-awareness, emotional problems related to difficulties adjusting to disability, social isolation and the like. By their very nature, none of these difficulties, not least problems of awareness and adjustment, are likely to respond to short-term episodes of psychological care. Much more likely is that it will probably take several sessions just to form a good understanding and mutually acceptable formulation of a given patient's presentation, suitable intervention, and outcome goals. The golden missing ingredient in all of this is . . . time. While some patients do derive some benefit from a specific short-term intervention (e.g. psycho-educational approaches in the early phases after acquired brain injury), many do not. We cannot let the Toms of this world leave as soon as a standard protocol has been delivered. For many, no good will come from such an approach.

4. Reflection

The truth of the matter in this example is that I went on to see the patient on whose case Tom is based, for many years. I also continued to regularly discuss him during my clinical supervision. One of the most significant early epochs in his therapy, described earlier, was when for the first time I had real empathy with his psychological struggle. I was perhaps (in an unsophisticated) way expressing my own frustration and sense of failure as a psychotherapist, after trying so hard to help Tom.

Reflecting on this experience, and my supervision at the time, is also a reminder that selection is by far the hardest part of clinical training. Yes, selection attempts to ascertain if short-listed applicants have the essential personal characteristics such as empathy, warmth, a genuine interest in others, compassion and the like. However, selection also considers very closely a person's ability to 'stay the course'. That is why selection is so hard. We can all run a qualifying time for participating in the marathon at the Olympic Games, if we were allowed to run 1 kilometre a week, and sum the individual times to submit as a 'qualifying time'. Selection (in most specialist professions and occupations) attempts to weed out applicants who give up too soon. Perhaps in a surprisingly compassionate way, selection acknowledges that clinical training, and making it your profession to see patients, is not for everyone.

In reality, I have had many Toms on my caseload. Returning to *this* Tom though, over time I learned many things about his unique difficulties. To some extent, with more time we discover our patients' unique psychological 'fingerprint' and accordingly update the neuropsychological formulation which drives their rehabilitation and psychotherapy. In Tom's case I gradually discovered that the cognitive impairment underpinning much of his agitation was related to very poor information processing, perhaps linked to poor attention. He simply could not understand what was being said. Unless a lot of time was invested, and sentences kept really short, he struggled to comprehend what was being communicated. In turn, this activated feelings (in CBT jargon, negative automatic thoughts) that threatened his sense of self: 'They think I am stupid!' Coupled with this, Tom also had the usual suite of executive difficulties: poor self-awareness, limited mental flexibility. In summary, he often retained little of what was said, and as a result became frustrated.

Let's now just have a look at Tom's difficulty with self-awareness. How can one begin CBT, or even consider compensatory strategies for poor recall, or commence psycho-education, if the patient does not acknowledge that these are problematic areas for them? The therapeutic relationship helps, as does credibility. But these are hard-earned commodities, requiring a considerable amount of patience, and time.

Now, add into all of this mix, the fact that every Tom brings with him (or her) a pre-morbid personality. As it turns out, Tom had some issues with a quick temper and impulsivity long before his injury. Well into our therapy, after he trusted me enough to talk about life before the injury, I was able to incorporate this into an updated formulation. But how would I have figured that out in ten sessions! As Pamela Klonoff so eloquently pointed out in her important book (2010) on psychotherapy in neurological populations: 'TTT' – things take time. Life in the trenches, of a daily clinical practice, working with unselected patients, whose problems are more severe than mild. That life is a bit different from the description in a research protocol.

References

Department of Health. (2005). *National service framework for long term neurological conditions*. London: Department of Health.

Klonoff, P. S. (2010). *Psychotherapy after brain injury. Principles and techniques*. New York: The Guilford Press.

Rogers, C. R. (1961). *On becoming a person*. Boston, MA: Houghton Mifflin.

14 This is not neuropsychological rehabilitation!

Christian Salas

'Theory is good, but it doesn't prevent things from existing'.

—Jean-Martin Charcot

1. Situation

There is something about professional training in clinical neuropsychology that is all about development and growth. We learn from supervisors, mentors and teachers about the world of neurological patients, how their minds change after damage to the brain, why they suffer and how we are supposed to help them. We learn to see through their eyes first, and only later, after many experiences and mistakes we manage to develop a personal point of view. Somehow, we inherit not only their knowledge and skills but also their blind spots. And their blind spots are the blind spots of their own supervisors and mentors. Like families, there are virtues and conflicts that can be passed from one generation of clinical neuropsychologists to another. When I was young, I was taught that neuropsychological rehabilitation was something we did *to* patients, to fix their minds, remediate their cognitive impairments, and heal their suffering. Now, almost decades later, I can see how naïve – and how omnipotent – that idea was. But everything is simpler and clearer in hindsight. My view of neuropsychological rehabilitation changed radically when I encountered an experience that completely challenged those beliefs. Something like those special moments during childhood, when you visit the home of a friend and realise that families can be so different, and house-rules so arbitrary.

2. Example

It was a long time ago. I was living in Manchester (UK) while writing up my PhD dissertation. Anyone who has gone through that process will tell you that it is a painful experience. Writing a thesis is like a marathon, a monotonous and tiresome endeavour, full of moments where you feel like giving up. It is not uncommon then to feel miserable and depressed. Honestly, humans are not made to write a PhD dissertation. It is unnatural. At that point, my dear wife told me I should do something about it. Probably I was making her life

DOI:10.4324/9781003300748-14

miserable too. So, she suggested that I should get out of the house and find something else to do besides sitting at home hitting the keyboard and moaning. One day she commented that there was this rehabilitation place in the city, a place for people with brain injuries, and that they accepted volunteers. So, I followed her advice, called the place and arranged a visit.

It is important to say that my experience of rehabilitation before Manchester was very medical. I worked for several years in a subacute rehabilitation hospital and an outpatient rehabilitation service in Chile (South America). Both places were run by rehabilitation doctors, so my job was basically to train cognitive functions, in the same way that a physical therapist trains a muscle to recover movement and strength. In my defence, I didn't know any better. Psychologists had a very peripheral role in those rehabilitation teams; patients had very few psychology hours, and we did not see patients in their natural environments. But that is how things were then, and still are in many services today! My colleagues and I had little formal training in neurorehabilitation, since clinical neuropsychology did not exist as a specialty at that time and there were no training programmes. So, nothing really prepared me for the huge surprise I received when arriving at the Head Forward Centre.[1] Perhaps in the same way that nothing could prepare an anthropologist that visits for the first time a distant and hidden civilisation.

If you passed quickly by the Withington Methodist Church, you would never guess what is going on at the back of such an old building. You had to really pay attention to realise that there is an iron gate at the side. A forgotten alley takes you to a door buried at the very end. Like in a story written by Lewis Carrol, a rusted and wet sign, with white and blue colours sits quietly next to the door, cryptically noting what is inside: Head Forward Centre. Later, I came to understand that this peculiar feeling I commonly experienced when arriving at Head Forward, the sensation of entering a place dislocated from the rest of the world, reflected a truth. Not many people knew the place. To say that is perhaps an understatement. Very few people and professionals knew this place existed. I can't help but think of one famous story by Asimov, where a group of scientists are secretly sent to the very edges of the galaxy to develop a new civilisation. Over the centuries, the colony is completely forgotten and abandoned to its faith, disconnected from the rest of the galaxy. I learnt many years later that the experience of isolation, the feeling of living in the margins of society, of not belonging to humanity, was a common experience amongst brain injury survivors.

I buzzed myself in. Soon a woman with a strong and beautiful Irish accent came to greet me. Her name was Maggie, and she was the manager of the place. Maggie was an English teacher, and her husband had a traumatic brain injury decades ago. We walked through a small hall and entered the main room. It is difficult to reconstruct my first impressions of the place since I later spent years living there, and Head Forward became a second home to me. And as you know, homes become a part of yourself, an extension of yourself. However, I do remember I was slightly disconcerted at first. Perhaps because the place did not fit into any pre-existent category I had of rehabilitation. I imagine that archaeologists feel the same way when they discover objects that do not resemble anything known. It is a strange mixture of perplexity and curiosity. The salon I entered was large with gigantic bright windows on one side. It had two pool tables in the middle which gave the whole room a beautiful and intense green glow. There were chairs all around and some tables where people ate, read the newspaper, or played dominoes. Some fellows were enthusiastically playing pool, teasing each other, while those looking from the side joined with comments and jokes. In the background a radio played old tunes: 'This is Smooth Radio'. From time to time, people began singing and dancing along to the music. When they realised Maggie and I were there, they waved and said hello, friendly but not really paying too much attention. And it is not that they didn't care, it is just that everyone was busy relaxing and enjoying themselves.[2]

My recollection of that day is not clear, but I remember that I spent the whole morning chatting, drinking tea and playing pool. Everyone was extremely friendly and sociable. They told me stories about their life and how this place helped them to feel less lonely and deal with the challenges of the outside world. By the end of that morning, I was over the moon and all my petty and bourgeois troubles about writing a thesis had vanished. I felt profoundly welcomed and curious about this particular place. So, when I was about to leave, Maggie asked me what I thought about the place. I remember that particular moment crystal clear. I said: what a wonderful rehabilitation service you have! Her look and reply to my words had marked my career for many years. She said, quickly trying to clarify something that I had apparently misunderstood: No, no, no . . . this is not a rehabilitation service. We do not do any assessment or cognitive retraining. We are a social rehabilitation facility. We only help them to socialise. I did not say anything back to her. While riding the bus back home, a feeling of perplexity lingered and Maggie's words kept resonating in my mind: this is not a rehabilitation service. As the bus moved towards the city centre I kept thinking, if this is not a rehabilitation service, what is it then?

3. Error

The error in this situation can be traced to the emotional reactions that Maggie and I experienced during that final word exchange. My surprise and perplexity suggested that Head Forward was something that did not fit into any of my preconceptions regarding how a rehabilitation service should be. The place was not run by doctors or rehabilitation professionals. The activities that took place there did not appear to target the common problems I was taught to represent the important issues of brain injury survivors.

None of my supervisors, and none of the books I had read, told me anything about this. These were truly unchartered waters. On the other hand, Maggie's emotional reaction reflected an even more problematic experience. Her quick and emphatic clarification suggested that considering Head Forward as a rehabilitation facility was a mistake, like an impostor that pretends to be something he is not. In her mind rehabilitation was something else, something more sophisticated, something done by professionals in medical contexts. If I can borrow a commonly used metaphor in psychoanalysis, 'traditional' or 'formal' rehabilitation was the *gold*, while Head Forward was something of lesser value, the copper. One can wonder where these ideas came from and how Maggie arrived at this view where social rehabilitation was less important than cognitive assessment and retraining.

I now believe that if I had presented, at that time, this dilemma to the people that attended HF, they would have laughed in my face saying I was talking nonsense. They would have said that this place was extremely important for their lives, providing an experience of normality, as well as social, emotional and cognitive support – in fact, these were all experiences that later on we managed to gather through in-depth interviews (Salas et al., 2021). In other words, the error here was that my neuropsychological rehabilitation knowledge and theory did not reflect reality, nor understood the psychological and social long-term needs of brain injury survivors. The problem in Maggie's response, what I have later come to think of as the 'ugly duckling' complex of social rehabilitation, is perhaps more challenging. Her conflicted experience probably reflected existing cultural beliefs about rehabilitation as a discipline; what it is and what is not, what are its goals, who can deliver interventions, etc. However, and in the same way that I had inherited beliefs about what patients need and what we are supposed to do to help them, Maggie had probably learnt these problematic views from her own experience as a brain injury carer and later as a service manager.

4. Reflection

As I mentioned before, getting to know Head Forward fundamentally changed the way I see neuropsychological rehabilitation. After that first visit, I began volunteering there and later was hired as a psychologist. How lucky I was! Since then, I became interested in what is termed informal rehabilitation, its therapeutic ingredients and relevance for long-term mental health outcomes. The term informal rehabilitation has been used to describe a wide range of initiatives including peer support groups, stroke clubs, Headway houses and other voluntary services. These services promote community integration and enhance social participation after hospital discharge, particularly during the chronic phase, when contact between rehabilitation professionals and patients/families is minimal. A main feature of informal rehabilitation is that it is often organised by people who live in the community and have some direct personal experience of brain damage and its ramifications (relatives, friends and 'expert' survivors). Peer-support groups like Head Forward are perhaps the best example of informal rehabilitation. In the UK, there are over 120 Headway groups and over 200 stroke groups or clubs. Surprisingly, if you look at any neuropsychological rehabilitation textbook this is still an extremely under-researched topic and we know little about how such interventions contribute to rehabilitation outcomes (for a review, see Hughes et al., 2020).

The lack of knowledge regarding the centrality of informal rehabilitation for community integration has profound implications. The most important one: we don't know how and why it works, thus compromising the possibility to improve this type of intervention and replicate it. As noted by Barbara Wilson (1997), we cannot rehabilitate without a theory of what needs to be rehabilitated. Together with Martin Cassassus, a friend and colleague from Chile who also worked at Head Forward, we have tried to address this theoretical challenge. Using in-depth interviews we found that years after the injury survivors experience high levels of social isolation, struggle to maintain old relationships and often are not able to develop new ones (Salas et al., 2018). We were also interested in the reasons why they attended Head Forward. So we asked them. Based on the data we gathered, a model of Social Rehabilitation was developed. This model proposed four key therapeutic ingredients: (a) provision of opportunities to stay socially and cognitive active; (b) provision of a network of continuous support; (c) provision of an environment that allows survivors to feel physically, emotionally and socially safe; (d) facilitate personal and social identity reconstruction (Salas et al., 2021). Later on, and using data from a sample of Chilean brain injury survivors who lived in the community, our research team explored the experience of loneliness and its relationship to mental health. We found that survivors who felt more lonely after the injury were likely to experience lower levels of quality of life and more depressive symptomatology (Salas et al., 2021). In conclusion, the phrase 'no man is an island' was particularly important to understand the complex long-term psychological needs of brain injury survivors.

I believe the data we have gathered can help overcome the 'ugly duckling' complex that exists in informal rehabilitation and perhaps modify the cultural beliefs that led Maggie to affirm that what they did at Head Forward was not rehabilitation. One of the main lessons I learnt at Head Forward was that perhaps this was the most important form of rehabilitation, one that helps survivors navigate their return to the community and regain a positive sense of self. Formal rehabilitation is with no doubt necessary, but its gains can easily disappear if survivors are not supported in facing the many challenges of living for years and decades with the consequences of a brain injury. As clinicians, we can support these initiatives in many ways. We can help colleagues and other rehabilitation professionals to become aware of the relevance of informal rehabilitation. We can educate survivors and relatives about the need to join these groups and collaborate in their formation. We can also gather evidence to justify the allocation of public and private resources to develop informal rehabilitation initiatives.

My take home message here is that there are many clinical situations where you will find that what we have been taught by our teachers or supervisors is insufficient, and that there are missing chapters in our rehabilitation books that still need to be written. Informal rehabilitation is only one of them. The same can apply to other relevant topics, such as changes in emotional or social life. But in order to write these chapters we need to follow Oliver Sacks' advice: visit our patients in the real world, leave our white coats and abandon our hospitals. We need to visit them and live for a season at the far borders of human experience.

Notes

1 www.headforward.org
2 You can have an idea of HeadForward by watching the documentary 'Personal Stories' made in collaboration with the Granada Centre for Visual Anthropology from Manchester University.

References

Hughes, R., Fleming, P., & Henshall, L. (2020). Peer support groups after acquired brain injury: A systematic review. *Brain Injury, 34*(7), 847–856.

Salas, C. E., Casassus, M., Rowlands, L., & Pimm, S. (2021). Developing a model of long-term social rehabilitation after traumatic brain injury: The case of the head forward centre. *Disability and Rehabilitation, 43*(23), 3405–3416.

Salas, C. E., Casassus, M., Rowlands, L., Pimm, S., & Flanagan, D. A. (2018). "Relating through sameness": A qualitative study of friendship and social isolation in chronic traumatic brain injury. *Neuropsychological Rehabilitation, 28*(7), 1161–1178.

Salas, C. E., Rojas-Líbano, D., Castro, O., Cruces, R., Evans, J., Radovic, D., . . . Aliaga, Á. (2021). Social isolation after acquired brain injury: Exploring the relationship between network size, functional support, loneliness and mental health. *Neuropsychological Rehabilitation, 32,* 2294–2318.

Wilson, B. A. (1997). Cognitive rehabilitation: How it is and how it might be. *Journal of the International Neuropsychological Society, 3*(5), 487–496.

15 Epilogue

Accepting and appreciating errors

Oliver Turnbull, Christian Salas & Rudi Coetzer

'I am glad that I paid so little attention to good advice; had I abided by it I might have been saved from some of my most valuable mistakes'.

—Edna St. Vincent Millay

The core of this book is a series of individual cases, and their associated mistakes. In this last chapter, we would like to frame the larger context of what *causes* errors. This is the most relevant aspect for clinical practice: discussing generic causes, the better to find generic solutions.

Mistakes, in the clinical domain, are a paradoxical combination: a mixture of the common and yet the rare. Mistakes are *common*, in that they happen quite often, especially to those who are early in their training, and presumably in any profession. There is an encouraging quote, from the physicist Niels Bohr, that 'An expert is a person who has made all the mistakes which can be made, in a narrow field'. One might debate the details, but the core of the observation is that there is no shame to making mistakes, not least because mistakes are potentially educational, and in the right hands can be a real learning opportunity.

However, we are left with the paradox: which is that mistakes are also rarely *reported*, presumably because of the feelings of shame and embarrassment that we associate with our failures. Of course, hiding failures from public view does not make mistakes unimportant. Critically, we can *avoid* making them in the future. Thus, it seems especially vital that we try, somehow, to discuss them, even if they do reflect uncomfortable truths. Making a mistake is no source of shame. Making the same mistake twice, however, is something quite different. And the best way to avoid 'twice' is to be aware of the first error, and to absorb its lesson.

Why mistakes happen?

Mistakes are caused, of course, for a variety of reasons. But it seems helpful to try and narrow down the likely causes of failure. These generic tips are especially helpful because an early career neuropsychologist is not likely to encounter the *precise* problems that we discuss in this book. You will make your own

DOI:10.4324/9781003300748-15

mistakes, and perhaps will tend to repeat some of them more than others. Your mistakes will have some features, but not all, in common with ours. Thus, we can use our examples to help you think about the likely causes of your mistakes, and to suggest helpful, broad-based, solutions.

This principle of generalisation is important, because our example errors provide only a few windows on to the field. Notably, the examples are from a fairly limited type of patient, which broadly reflects our training on adult neurology and neurosurgery wards, and in adult brain injury reha-bilitation units. There are entire categories of neuropsychological disorder and neurological disease that are not much present in the book. We have many cases of closed head injury and stroke, but no examples from (say) dementia or paediatric neuropsychology, nothing from anterior temporal lobectomy, or toxic/metabolic conditions. But we are not here to work our way through a neurology textbook, rather to show examples of *how* think-ing can go awry. We seek to illustrate general principles, rather than specific skills, and to develop an attitude towards errors that can promote learning from experience.

What, then, and might be those principles that underpin errors? And what might the solutions be?

1. *Grow your knowledge base*

The greatest challenge for trainees in clinical neuropsychology comes, natu-rally, from the fact that the field is so complex, and is complex in a number of ways. Perhaps the most daunting is that clinical neuropsychology is surrounded by other disciplines, each of which, on its own, represents a large domain of enquiry. For example, there is no clinical neuropsychology without an under-standing of neuroanatomy: from the caudate to the cortex; and from the ven-tricles to the vascular system, neuroanatomy is an entire field of study. The early career clinical neuropsychologist must master neuroanatomy, at least the level of a generalist medical student.

Actually, the level of a medical student is not going to be good enough, because the trainee clinical neuropsychologist is not going to *meet* many medi-cal students. They will meet neurologists, neurosurgeons, or more likely their Registrars or House officers, whose training requires them to know anatomy in impressive detail: blood supply to the basal ganglia; likely sites of aneurysm rupture in the Circle of Willis; origin and course of the cranial nerves. These are entry-level anatomy facts for a neurologist or neurosurgeon,[1] but hard-won knowledge for a trainee clinical neuropsychologist.

And yet, this is only *one* of the surrounding fields. The aspiring neuropsy-chologist also needs to know something of, naturally, neurology,[2] of neuro-pathology, of neuroradiology, of basic statistics, and indeed of psychiatry and clinical psychology. Examples of errors that follow from poor knowledge of these fields, and the challenges of integrating these diverse sources of informa-tion, are dotted across this book. So, as it must be for *any* trainee, there seems far too much to know. Indeed, if the early career clinician isn't careful, they will think that they don't know *anything*, and this chapter aims to protect you against some of those feelings.

One saving grace is that the trainee's *formal* course should (at least in locations where there *are* formal courses) cover the bare bones of this material. Nevertheless, a risk arises because there is a difference between covering material in a lecture or exam, and the sort of familiarity that comes with repeated exposure. Fluency takes time, and can be intimidating when the learner encounters it. A terrifying element of the 'surrounding disciplines' problem is joining a team of specialists, who already know the field incredibly well. Your multidisciplinary team may already seem like a tidy family unit, chattering away in a language of shared knowledge and secret acronyms. On a bad day, the MDT (if we are speaking of acronyms) may automatically assume that their terminology is already understood by the trainee. Much of their communication will seem cryptic, and their confidence can be daunting.

So, what to do when you don't know something? Is a Grade 4 glioma good or bad news? A GCS of 10? What does it mean when the patient's notes say NIDDM, or WNL? Can you just ask someone? In one sense, yes, you can: explain that you don't have the first idea what they are talking about, and hope that the professional will give you a brief tutorial. In our experience, this is a card that you can play only occasionally, because these are busy people, and they may not feel that they have time to explain what has seemed obvious to them for years.

An alternative, which we would highly recommend, is to write down the details that you don't understand (perhaps even phonetically?), and then furiously try to catch up later. Make friends. Ask someone that you can trust after the meeting. Having the internet at your fingertips is clearly also a real help. Gradually, the terminology will become familiar, and slowly your colleagues will no longer sound as if they are talking in a foreign language.

In summary, many of your errors will come from lack of knowledge, in a field (or fields) where there is a lot to learn. The best advice is to accept not only that the challenge is substantial but also that it can be overcome by gradually working on all of the gaps in your knowledge. A century of memory research tells us that regular practice beats binge study, and that learning is always more complete when it is 'deep', or embedded in a broader semantic network. A case-based approach can be the way forward to integrate new knowledge into your growing 'clinical neuropsychology' semantic network. Don't try and read the neuropathology book cover to cover. But when you meet a colloid cyst, or a meningioma, for the first time, *that* is the moment to read the relevant chapter. Probably twice. Your knowledge of the third ventricle, and the consequences of CSF blockage, will now always be linked to your first case of a colloid cyst. And tomorrow, you will meet a patient who had a posterior cerebral artery aneurysm, and *that* will be the moment to remind yourself about the Circle of Willis. Each patient is a new chapter to read. Small steps, every day, and you will travel a long way.

2. No piece is the whole jigsaw

Reaching a conclusion, a formulation, about a patient is an exercise in pulling together information from radically different sources. Perhaps the most obvious failure, and a common source of error, is a tendency to over-rely in one source or type of information. We have several examples of 'jigsaw puzzle' errors in this book, and an extremely common error is to exclusively rely on psychological test results (see our chapter on why these are not *neuro*psychological test results). Why is this error type common? Perhaps because the formal test is the most respectable sounding piece of equipment in the neuropsychologist's tool kit. Tests give you a score, the norms will tell you whether the patient has 'passed' or 'failed', and in the manual, there will be details of which cognitive ability or psychological process may be impaired.

Alas, tests can be remarkably imprecise. Our chapters show the several ways that they can be misleading. Most notably, it is surprisingly easy to fail a psychological test. In one of our examples, a patient does badly for psychiatric reasons. In another, the patient does *have* a brain lesion, but un-sportingly fails for reasons that aren't the ones described in the manual. Patients often perform worse (or better) than expected, for reasons related to their premorbid capacities and personality traits, cultural or educational background, their social class, or even their hobbies and careers. One of our examples is a patient who wasn't really *trying* to pass the test . . . or perhaps was trying *not* to pass the test? In another of our examples, the patient does better than they should, because the neuropsychologist wasn't assessing the patient *at all*! And then there's the question of whether the neuropsychologist is administering the *correct* test? Choosing the right test, and making sure that the patient is given the best chance to perform on it, is far more important than the apparently satisfying act of scoring the measure. As our colleague Mark Solms put it (and actually quoting Mike Saling): 'the psychometric approach to neuropsychology was so popular because it was so easy' (Coetzer & Balchin, 2014, p. xi).

A football analogy might be useful here. Administering the tests can be compared to the process of kicking the ball into the back of the net. Of scoring the goal, when you are *already in* the penalty area. Now, scoring the goal is important, but the really hard work was done earlier, by moving the ball down the pitch, and into the penalty area in the first place. In this analogy, that vital *preparatory* work is done by a range of pieces of information, *none* of which involve psychological *tests* at all.

This preparation comes from taking a sound history from the patient, and from family or friends if possible. Another strand is to consider this in the context of their medical history, and also the patient's life circumstances. Ideally, we are looking for all this information to align: the lesion site, the time course of the disease, the type of deficit reported by the patient and the family, and indeed the way that the patient reports the problem when you take the history. In a sense, we are asking which neuropsychological impairment the patient is 'entitled' to (Walsh, 1985). A patient is 'entitled' to a problem when a known pathological process produces a lesion in a known location, when the disorder has progressed at a rate consistent with this disease type, where the patient and family report problems consistent with this lesion site, and where the patient *behaves* (in the clinic *and* outside it) in a manner consistent with that neuropsychological disorder. All the elements are aligned.

When this information *does* align, then your tests are often, or ideally, administered in order to *confirm* this conclusion, to measure the *extent* of the impairment with more precision, to see whether the patient performs in the way that you might expect them to, based on the hypothesis you have built up, as you moved the ball down the football pitch. This is one of the reasons that Walsh uses the, earlier cited, and devastating, phrase that there is no such thing as a neuropsychological test. There are too many ways to 'fail' a psychological test, and a test tells you very little out of context. The test result can seem such a tempting, simple answer. But no jigsaw piece is the whole puzzle. All, or at least most, of the pieces need to fit together before we have the answer.

Many of the mistakes in the book take this form. As you have seen, they are often examples where *some* elements of the case led us in one direction, and we were dazzled by this. However, we then chose to *ignore* other elements of the case, which later turned out to be inconvenient truths. So, the second way to avoid mistakes is remembering to view the patient's case in the round. Look for converging evidence, not single facts. Do all the elements of the jigsaw puzzle align? Are there parts that don't make sense? When you reach this point, then test performance is just the final confirmation of a pattern that already made sense.

3. Step back, and look at the big picture. Develop your intuition

This then begs the question of what you should do when the pattern *doesn't* make sense. Our recommendation here is to get some perspective, to give yourself some time, to rethink things, to do some reading, and to ask someone experienced for advice. There is a reason that those detective programmes on television last for a whole hour, and not just for 10 minutes. To Miss Marple or Inspector Morse, the answer may look quite obvious early on in the mystery, but our heroine or hero steps away from the problem, because there is something that just doesn't make sense. *Most* of the case seems to fit together, but our detective is worried by an inconsistency.

As a neuropsychologist, this is a situation well worth being aware of. Perhaps the history didn't match the test performance? Perhaps the patient's account doesn't fit that of the family. Or, considering the patient's background, they did remarkably well, or remarkably poorly, on this or that sort of test? This is a great moment for a neuropsychologist to give themselves some time to reconsider. To go and read a book, or ask a colleague. Or take a walk in the hospital garden, have your lunch, talk to the hospital porter about their family, or the weather, to get a sense of perspective. Give yourself the luxury of a little time, if you have it – and especially, to go back and look at the *evidence* again.

Many of the examples in this book derive from situations that would have benefited from a good night's sleep, or talking the case over with someone – or perhaps even just talking the case over with *oneself*. Across our careers, we have often found it helpful to just talk through the fundamentals of the case with somebody knowledgeable, or even just to have some form of self-talk. Does everything align? What are the causes of doubt? Is there an alternative account?

Notably, you can weigh up whether any element of the evidence might be unreliable? Was the patient having a bad day when they were tested? Had the family left out a critical source of information? Does this disease process sometimes manifest in unusual ways? What then? If possible, allow yourself the opportunity to do what happens in all those detective films: to go back and gather more evidence. A lovely moment often happens when the detective (especially Columbo) is *about* to leave the room, and then says: 'Just one more thing', before asking a critical question. More information, and a fresh look at things, can be really valuable. For example, to see the same patient on a different day, to ask them a different set of questions, to see them perform a parallel version of the test, or a different test which is supposed to measure the same underlying skill. You may be surprised at the extent to which patients can present in different ways under these altered circumstances.

Critically, there should be no sense of shame or embarrassment in gathering this extra information. In the chapters of this book, we have often framed this reassessment phase as happening after an embarrassing moment with the supervisor.[3] But this need not be the case. You can short-circuit the process that leads to an embarrassing outcome by presenting the case to a trusted colleague, or indeed just to yourself. You'll be surprised how much you can learn from looking at things for a second time, or in a new light?

Critically, this process of revaluation can lead to the development of an entirely different hypothesis. Perhaps a known pathological process produced damage to an unexpected brain area? Perhaps the poor test performance is not from loss of a foundational skill, but a failure of executive function – or alternatively, not a failure of executive function, but just the absence of a simple foundational skill. Several of this book's chapters take this general form: Assessment of something that seems clear, then a reflection and reconsideration, leading to a new hypothesis about the nature of the patient's impairment. To continue the football analogy, it is now a different player dribbling the ball down the pitch, and we may need a different set of psychological tests in order to confirm or disprove the hypothesis.

Knowing that you are *able* to reconsider the case, that you're allowed to change your mind, is a critical skill, which we hope this book has helped you to develop. This freedom will allow you to carry on thinking about your patients long after you have finished an initial assessment, and to feel no sense of shame about developing and then testing different hypotheses. Critically, this process will also help to develop a sense of intuition about *when* you can be confident in your judgement, and when you should be more sceptical. This process of 'intuition' is a well-known neuropsychological phenomenon, on which one of us has published a few papers on over the years (Turnbull, 2003; Turnbull et al., 2005, 2007, 2014). More accurately described as 'emotion-based learning' (Turnbull et al., 2005), intuition follows from repeated exposure to complex problems, and learning (implicitly) from the emotional consequences of the outcomes. *This* is why Kevin Walsh is commonly cited as using the phrase that: 'Neuropsychology is a body contact sport'.[4] You need to see real patients, on which you will sometimes reach inaccurate conclusions. And if, or more likely *when*, you fail, you will learn from your mistakes. This will hurt. But it will be worth the pain.

In this sense, then, mistakes are a critically important part of the learning process. Because, after some learning has occurred, you can develop an awareness of an *impending* error, and protect you from the consequences of reaching the wrong conclusion in future. The critical word in the last sentence is 'awareness'. It is one thing to give yourself time to consider the case, but it's another entirely to have some *awareness* that you may be sitting on a mistake of one kind or another. This is that sense of intuition (or gut feeling) which is often described by experts in their field. Something feels wrong, even though they can't describe formally what the cause of the problem is. Intuition (or emotion-based learning) is not, of course, something supernatural, and is increasingly better understood. It appears to be a form of acquired knowledge or emotion-based skill.

Furthermore, clinicians often exhibit patterns of mistakes that tend to repeat in time. These are related to personality traits, to what and how they have learnt from other clinicians, and to counter-transferential feelings towards patients, supervisors and themselves. Just like a chess player, clinicians can systematically err in their openings, middle game, or endings (Soltis, 1979). Becoming aware of these patterns can help you to detect them in advance, and find an alternative course of action.

Two points seem relevant in relation to the question of errors and emotion-based learning. The first of them is that the skill is acquired based on *feelings*. It is about having a number of attempts at a problem, some of them ending well and others badly, and then (implicitly) learning patterns of association between our actions and their emotional consequences. Thus, if the trainee is not making mistakes, if they are not sometimes feeling bad, then they're not acquiring the (implicit) knowledge needed to improve. In that sense, mistakes are good, because they are foundational to learning. The flip side is that we need to catch the mistakes, and contain them, before they negatively impact on patients. This is the purpose, of course, of supervision. The good supervisor (gently) shows you the mistake, and prevents its consequences from interfering with the treatment process. So don't kick yourself for making mistakes. They are a valuable part of skill acquisition. However, we are surprised at how little space has been dedicated to mistakes in the supervision literature. Feedback to clinical neuropsychology trainees, and correcting errors, has been repeatedly described as central for the supervision process (Stucky et al., 2010). Yet mistakes are not a common topic of discussion during supervision (Shultz et al., 2014).

The second point is that the acquisition of the skill takes time. It is based on the gradual accumulation of the emotional consequences of ideas, so that we are able to run a thought experiment, or a trial action, to consider how things in the future will pan out. Neuropsychology is therefore not merely a body contact sport, as we suggested, but a sport which requires extensive practice in order to improve.

We hope you have enjoyed these painful reminders, a re-exploring of the errors that we made in our earlier years, but can also remerge later in our careers. They represent hard-won knowledge, sometimes associated with feelings of shame, but feelings which we have now come to terms with. We hope that you, too, are able to accept your mistakes in a positive light.

Notes

1 Here is a salutary quote from Mark Solms (Coetzer & Balchin, 2014, p. x) on his initial encounter with the clinical world:

> It was clear to me that this neurosurgeon assumed I knew things that I had never even heard of before. He talked a language that was entirely foreign to me, not only in its obscure technical terminology but also the whole worldview upon which rested. There was a hidden order to his thinking, completely obscure to me, with all sort of assumptions about what is and is not relevant . . . about all of which I knew next to nothing.

Admittedly, Solms' situation was unusual, and reflects the 'under-resourced settings' of the Coetzer and Balchin (2014) book. In passing, Solms' Foreword to that book makes fascinating reading for a modern trainee, who will thank their lucky stars if they have received a more formal and supported introduction to the clinical world.
2 In our Preface, we spoke of Kevin Walsh aphorisms, as his way of summarising key truths in the field. Walsh himself (1992, p. 120) cites Peter Bladin in a classic gnome: 'No neuropsychology without neurology'.
3 Here is a reminder, as we discussed in Chapter 1, that we have used for a certain amount of artistic licence in these descriptions, to preserve patient and supervisor anonymity.
4 This is an aphorism commonly linked to Walsh, but he himself attributes it to Peter Bladin (Walsh, 1992, p. 123).

References

Coetzer, R., & Balchin, R. (2014). *Working with brain injury: A primer for psychologists working in under-resourced settings*. London: Psychology Press.
Shultz, L. A. S., Pedersen, H. A., Roper, B. L., & Rey-Casserly, C. (2014). Supervision in neuropsychological assessment: A survey of training, practices, and perspectives of supervisors. *The Clinical Neuropsychologist, 28*(6), 907–925.
Soltis, A. (1979). *Catalog of chess mistakes*. New York: D. McKay Company.
Stucky, K. J., Bush, S., & Donders, J. (2010). Providing effective supervision in clinical neuropsychology. *The Clinical Neuropsychologist, 24*(5), 737–758.
Turnbull, O. H. (2003). Emotion, false beliefs, and the neurobiology of intuition. In J. Corrigall & H. Wilkinson (Eds.), *Revolutionary connections: Psychotherapy and neuroscience* (pp. 135–162). London: Karnac Books.

Turnbull, O. H., Bowman, C. H., Shanker, S., & Davies, J. L. (2014). Emotion-based learning: Insights from the Iowa Gambling Task. *Frontiers of Psychology*, *5*(Article 162): 1–11. doi: 10.3389/fpsyg.2014.00162

Turnbull, O. H., Evans, C. E. Y., Bunce, A., Carzolio, B., & O'Connor, J. (2005). Emotion-based learning and central executive resources: An investigation of intuition and the Iowa Gambling Task. *Brain and Cognition*, *57*, 244.

Turnbull, O. H., Worsey, R., & Bowman, C. H. (2007). Emotion and intuition: Does *schadenfreude* make interns poor learners? *Philoctetes*, *1*, 5–43.

Walsh, K. W. (1985). *Understanding brain damage: A primer of neuropsychological evaluation*. Edinburgh: Churchill Livingstone.

Walsh, K. (1992). Some gnomes worth knowing. Clinical Neuropsychologist, 6(2), 119–133. https://doi.org/10.1080/13854049208401849

Index